Psychoactive Drugs and Sex

Psychoactive Drugs and Sex

Ernest L. Abel

Springer Science+Business Media, LLC

Library of Congress Cataloging in Publication Data

Abel, Ernest L., 1943–
  Psychoactive drugs and sex.

  Includes bibliographies and index.
  1. Generative organs—Effect of drugs on. 2. Psychotropic drugs—Physiological effect.
3. Drugs and sex. I. Title. [DNLM: 1. Psychotropic Drugs—pharmacodynamics. 2. Sex. 3.
Sex Behavior—drug effects. QV 77 A139p]
RM380.A24   1985   615′.788   84-26446

ISBN 978-1-4899-3640-0   ISBN 978-1-4899-3638-7 (eBook)
DOI 10.1007/978-1-4899-3638-7

© 1985 Springer Science+Business Media New York
Originally published by Plenum Press, New York in 1985.
Softcover reprint of the hardcover 1st edition 1985

Contents

Introduction

The search for artificial means of enhancing sexual experience is timeless and can even be found in the opening passages of Genesis (3:7) where Adam and Eve discovered sex as they took a bite of the forbidden fruit: "And the eyes of them both were opened, and they knew that they were naked." While others may interpret the "opening of their eyes" as simply an awareness of male and femaleness, John Milton and others regarded the forbidden fruit as an aphrodisiac and in *Paradise Lost*, described in greater detail what happened:

> "But the false fruit
> For other operation first displayed
> Carnal desire inflaming. He on Eve
> Began to cast lascivious eyes; she him
> As wantonly repaid; in lust they burn."

Not only did Milton regard the "forbidden fruit" as an aphrodisiac, he also identified it as an apple, and an apple it has remained until this day.

Sexual behavior has always been one of the most fascinating and attention-arresting activities in human history and there has been no decrease in the fascination and curiosity it still arouses in the human psyche.

1

As timeless as the topic of sexual behavior is that of aphrodisiacs. For example, after the "forbidden fruit," the Bible specifically identified mandrake as an aphrodisiac (Genesis 30:14–17):

> "And Reuben went, in the days of wheat harvest, and found mandrakes in the field, and brought them to his mother, Leah. Then Rachel said to Leah, Give me, I pray thee, of thy son's mandrake.
> And she said unto her. It is a small matter that thou hast taken my husband? and wouldest thou take away my son's mandrakes also? And Rachel said, Therefore he shall be with thee to-night for thy son's mandrakes.
> And Jacob came out of the field in the evening, and Leah went out to meet him, and said, Thou must come in unto me, for surely I have hired thee with my son's mandrakes. And he lay with her that night.
> And God hearkened unto Leah, and she conceived, and bore Jacob, the fifth son."

Alongside the ancient Hebrews, the Babylonians and Egyptians were also preoccupied with discovering and using substances that would increase sexual desire or potency, or enhance sexual performance. The term aphrodisiac itself comes from Aphrodite, the Greek goddess of love. According to Greek mythology, she arose from the sea and bestowed sexual enjoyment on mankind. Whereas the cult of Aphrodite did not survive the centuries, the search for aphrodisiacs has continued up until the present and shows no sign of abating.

Whatever their source, aphrodisiacs are generally taken to increase sexual arousal or to enhance sexual performance. Although enhanced sexuality is usually the goal of people seeking to change their sexuality, in some cases decreases in sexual arousal are sought. The search for such "anaphrodisiacs" was usually to help people break free of romantic involvements. In some cases, these substances were also sought after by those trying to preserve their chastity. Monks, for example, grew rue, "the herb of grace," in their monastic gardens to dampen their arousal. Nuns, however, stayed away from the same plant because it was supposed to have an opposite effect in women. Instead of rue, they ate water lily to help them get over any feelings or acts that would damn their souls. Today there is very little demand for anaphrodisiacs. One exception is in the case of sexual offenders who sometimes agree to take drugs such as the antiandrogen, cyproterone, to decrease sexual arousal.

Many illicit drugs are still taken for the express purpose of affecting sexual arousal or performance. Therapeutic drugs taken for sanctioned purposes may also have unwanted sexual effects. Usually, these unwanted effects involve decreased rather than enhanced function, such as loss of libido, erectile dysfunction or ejaculatory failure in the male, and inability to achieve orgasm in the female. Although such effects are noted in manuals such as the *Physician's Desk Reference*, just as they were noted in the pharmacopoeas of the last century, there are few books that deal with such relations in any depth.

This book describes sexually-related effects of illicit, social, and therapeutic drugs. In contrast to therapeutic drugs that are taken for specific medical reasons, illicit and social drugs are taken for nonmedical reasons, usually for their effects on "consciousness."

In most cases, it is impossible to assess objectively the claims made about any drug's effect on sexual arousal or performance. This is simply because experiments involving human sexual activity and drugs are not countenanced. In some cases, there have been studies of drugs on sexual function, but these are few and far between. Studies of sexual activity in animals can often provide insights into possible human activities, but apart from the basic problem of extrapolation from animals to humans, there are also basic methodological problems, e.g., drug dosage, that must be considered. Another reason for the difficulty in evaluating reports of sexual effects is that descriptions of these effects are often vague. For example, male impotence is often rated as a side effect of drugs, but the nature of this impotence is not described, e.g., loss of libido, erectile failure.

BASIC CONSIDERATIONS

To evaluate the potential effects of any drug as a sexual stimulant or depressant, it is important to take into account both that drug's pharmacology, the individual using it, and the circumstances or conditions at time of use.

Pharmacological Factors

With respect to pharmacological factors, the amount of drug taken (dose-response), the route of administration (i.v., oral), previous experience with the drug ("tolerance"), and other drugs of the same class ("cross-tolerance") are as important as the drug itself. If so little of the drug is taken that it is incapable of causing any effect, then it is obviously impossible to evaluate. Similarly, if so much of the drug is taken that it produces sedation or unconsciousness, then other possible effects will not be seen. The time lapsing between drug taking and a particular behavior is equally important. If a drug is taken one day and some event takes place the next, the likelihood of the drug causing or contributing to that event is much lower than if the event occurred soon after the drug was taken.

The route of administration by which a drug is introduced into the body may affect its perceived effects. Typically drugs such as heroin or methamphetamine produce a "rush" or elation which has been compared to an orgasm, when these drugs are administered intravenously. Part of this orgasmic reaction may include the act of intravenous administration per se since many of those who inject themselves intravenously report orgasmic reactions from simply administering water. The symbolism between the needle and the penis has also been commented upon in this regard.

Familiarity with a particular drug will also affect reaction to it. Knowing what to expect and being prepared for it is included in the term "set." If one is "set" to experience excitation and a drug produces depression, then confusion may mask drug effects such as aphrodisia. Experience with a drug, particularly chronic habitual experience, may result in "tolerance." This means that more of the same drug will have to be used to produce the same effect as was initially experienced when the drug was first used. Alternatively, tolerance can be defined in terms of the same amount of drug producing a smaller effect than that originally produced as a result of chronic usage. Cross-tolerance is a related phenomenon. This refers to experience with one drug conveying tolerance to another, even if the second has never been used. Cross-tolerance occurs between alcohol and barbiturate drugs, for example. Chronic use of a drug over an intense period (a "run") may also result in physical exhaustion so that possible stimulation will be masked.

Individual Factors

The individual using a particular drug is a second major factor determining whether a drug will have sexual effects (or whether sexual effects will be reported). Individuals who are shy and inhibited may benefit from using drugs which decrease such personality traits. This is one of the reasons alcohol has been touted as a sexual stimulant through the ages since it enhances interpersonal relations for many. Amphetamines may also give one more confidence as part of their overall excitatory effects and this too may be perceived in specific rather than general terms.

In some cases, enhancement of drug effects may lack any objective basis. For example, Freedman (1976) describes the case of an individual who perceived a need to improve his sexual competence and believed he had achieved improvement via amyl nitrite:

> "One young man claimed that when he crushed a vial of amyl nitrite just before having an orgasm, his experience was extraordinary, better than his experiences with any other drugs. However, when he was closely questioned, it became clear that he was so preoccupied with crushing the capsule at the right moment and sniffing the vapor, thereby altering his mental state, that he was scarcely aware of what really happened".

Another important consideration from the standpoint of the individual is related to the previous level of sexual activity. A drug is much more likely to increase libido and sexual behavior if these occur infrequently than at a higher level. Similarly, a drug is more likely to decrease libido and sexual activity when these already occur with a relatively high frequency. This is because in the first case, there is little opportunity for sexual activity to decrease any further whereas in the second case, further increases may not be physically or socially possible. This dependence on pre-existing levels of behavior is sometimes considered in terms of "rate dependence." A second individual factor that has already been mentioned is "set." This refers to the individual's expectations or anticipations concerning drug effects. Gay and Sheppard (1972) quote one of their respondents in this regard: "I dig sex on uppers, downers, drugs that take me sideways, and those that turn me inside-out. Even a placebo would probably sex me up if I thought it would alter me in some way."

Conditions at Time of Use

The social context in which drug effects are experienced is the third major factor contributing to possible drug effects on libido and sexual activity. Obviously, if one is in the midst of battle, drug effects on libido or sexual behavior are unlikely to manifest themselves. This is why reports of sexual effects were not associated with amphetamines among soldiers in battle. Similarly, while a drug may increase libido, the possibility that this increase will be expressed depends on the behavior of others.

Apart from these basic pharmacological, personal, and social considerations, there is another basic consideration which involves a willingness to discuss sex. For example, in cases where drugs are used for therapeutic purposes some patients may be reluctant to discuss changes in sexuality associated with drug use. This reluctance to discuss sexual side effects may result in considerable underreporting.

DEFINITIONS

Aphrodisiacs are generally regarded as substances that enhance libido or sexual function. Most assessments of claims for aphrodisiacal properties of drugs have concluded that any claims for enhanced sexuality are due to nonspecific effects such as reduction in inhibitions or general stimulation. Most efforts to identify aphrodisiacs have generally been dismissed as failures due to the emphasis on these two criteria (Gawin, 1978). If however, increased sexual pleasure is included as a criterion, more drugs may become recognized for their aphrodisiac properties.

Gawin (1978) considers the standard definition of aphrodisiacs too narrow and proposes an expanded definition to include "an effect of a pharmacological substance on the subjective pleasure of sexual experience, independent of any effect at all on what is commonly considered libido or sexual drive". This definition, Gawin (1978) argues, presumes the pre-existence of libido. Aphrodisiacs are therefore substances which enhance rather than initiate sexual experience. Gawin's definition also seems narrow, but the inclusion of sexual pleasure is an important one. A revision of the definition of aphrodisiacs is one describing them as substances that enhance libido, sexual function, or sexual enjoyment.

Sexual Arousal generally refers to sexual desire or libido. It is a subjective response which may or may not be associated with objective responses such as penile erection in the male or increased vaginal flow in the female. Lack of interest or sexual inhibitions are included under the category of sexual arousal since such problems can be differentiated from functional disorders which may occur in individuals who are sexually interested.

Sexual arousal depends on a complex interaction between individual, social, and cultural factors. A lot depends on experience, and on the individual's general state of sexual arousal. In many cases, sexual dysfunction may be due to individual factors arising out of early sexual experiences that caused guilt or anxiety, or to lack of information, or to situational factors such as job-related factors or marital stress. Such problems may be treated with psychotherapy or with anti-anxiety drugs.

Sexual arousal and function are related to hormonal function. Some drugs may affect sexuality by altering the production or release of hormones or by affecting the delicate feedback mechanisms that regulate hormonal levels in the body. Testosterone's role in sexuality is the best known and most carefully studied thus far.

In the male, testosterone is produced by the Leydig cells in the testes, in response to luteinizing hormone (LH) released from the anterior pituitary. Release of this pituitary hormone is controlled by the hypothalamus through hypothalamic LH-releasing hormone (LH-RH). Spermatogenesis is controlled by another pituitary hormone, FSH. In the female, ovulation is also controlled by LH and FSH.

Testosterone levels in the blood are monitored by the hypothalamus in a negative hypothalamic-pituitary-gonadal feedback axis such that high levels cause the hypothalamus to decrease production of hormones that stimulate the pituitary whereas low levels cause it to stimulate the pituitary. Decreased testosterone levels could thus be due to decreased release of hypothalmic LH-RH, decreased responsiveness of the pituitary to LH-RH (decreased LH secretion by the pituitary), decreased responsiveness of the Leydig cells to LH, Leydig cell damage, or decreased sensitivity of the hypothalamus to testosterone.

Evidence for testosterone's contribution to sexual arousal comes from studies in men and animals showing that sexual arousal generally decreases after castration. Similarly, anti-androgen drugs such as cyproterone acetate which block the actions of testosterone in the brain and lower plasma testosterone levels decrease sexual arousal. These changes do not occur immediately. The decrease in sexual arousal resulting from cyproterone for example, does not appear until about two weeks after drug therapy is begun and does not stop until about two weeks after therapy is discontinued.

Testosterone is also the major hormone that affects sexual arousal in women. Decreases in testosterone levels in women caused by removal of the adrenals (the main source of testosterone in women) decreases sexual arousal whereas administration of testosterone increases sexual arousal in women (Carney *et al.*, 1978). Estrogens, the main hormones produced by the ovaries, are important for vaginal lubrication. Controlled studies in women using the "pill" indicate that these drugs do not affect sexual arousal per se but may affect expectations which then result in either increased or decreased arousal (Bragonier, 1976).

In most cases, however, testosterone only seems to affect sexual arousal when there is an initial sexual dysfunction. In the absence of sexual dysfunction testosterone does not affect sexual arousal.

In men, feminization and hypogonadism are often associated with increased clearance of testosterone and decreased clearance of estrogens. The latter may be due to resorption of estrogens into the blood due to liver disease. To the extent that male libido is affected by the balance between male and female sex steroid levels, drug-related effects on such steroids will affect male libido whether drugs act directly on the testes or indirectly on mechanisms related to testes function.

Direct evidence that drugs inhibit Leydig cell function comes from *in vitro* studies in which testosterone production by Leydig cells is first stimulated by chorionic gonadotropin or cyclic AMP and after which the experiment is repeated in the presence of various drugs.

Sexual Behavior refers to behavior connected with sexual activity. This may take the form of masturbation or sexual intercourse. In some studies, the definition of sexual behavior has been broadened to include sexual thoughts as well.

Sexual behavior has been most thoroughly studied in animals, especially rodents, and involves a complicated interplay of events. Although the relation of such studies to human activity is often unclear, studies in animals offer insights into possible neurochemical mechanisms that may mediate sexual activity in both animals and humans.

Sexual Function refers to the mechanical aspects of sexual activity such as penile erection or vaginal lubrication. Various dysfunctions include erectile failure and premature ejaculation in the male or decreased vaginal lubrication or vaginismus in the female.

Penile erection can originate centrally from neural impulses arising in the brain and descending through the spine to the autonomic nervous system, or can be a reflex response to tactile stimulation of the genital area.

As described by Masters and Johnson (1966) sexual function

can be divided into four main phases in both men and women. These phases are not clearly separated from one another, but provide a useful model for examining sexual function.

1. Excitement Phase. Sexual excitement may be either physical or psychic in origin. In the male, this is associated with penile vasocongestion and erection.

Neural activity originating in cortical and limbic centers of the brain (presumably "primed" by testosterone) initiates efferent activity in sympathetic and parasympathetic neurons to initiate or inhibit penile tumescence. Tumescence can also be produced reflexively by tactual stimulation of the genitals (Kuhn, 1950).

Penile erection occurs as a result of vasodilation leading to engorgement of erectile tissues by blood. Such engorgement is normally prevented by sympathetic and parasympathetic impulses to "polsters" which restrict blood flow into the penis. Sexual arousal causes relaxation of the "polsters," thus permitting entry of blood. Ejaculation is controlled by reflex mechanisms located in the second and third lumbar region. Stimulation of these areas initiates contraction of the seminal vesicles, the vas deferens, and the bulbar muscles, resulting in ejaculation. Penile erection is mainly controlled by the cholinergically-mediated parasympathetic system whereas ejaculation is primarily mediated by the adrenergically-mediated sympathetic system (see below).

Studies in animals using electrodes implanted in various parts of the brain have shown the existence of excitatory centers for erection in the limbic system and inhibitory centers in the thalamus (Maclean, 1976). These centers send impulses through the spinal cord to erectile mechanisms. Transection of the spinal cord above the sacral level will eliminate all central influences on erection but will not affect reflex erection (Kuhn, 1950).

In the female, sexual excitation is associated with labial and vulvar vasocongestion, vaginal lubrication and swelling, increase in clitoral size, and erection of the nipples. Clitoral arousal results from parasympathetic stimulation whereas orgasm results from sympathetic stimulation. Since sexual responsiveness is mediated by the autonomic nervous system, drugs that affect this system may thus have a direct effect on sexual function.

2. Plateau Phase. In the male, this phase is associated with maximal penile engorgement and is accompanied by secretion of the Cowper's gland. In the female, this is associated with maximal vaginal swelling and elevation of the uterus.

3. Orgasm. This is associated with ejaculation in the male. Ejaculation is caused by reflex mechanisms located in the second and third lumbar spinal region. Stimulation of these areas causes involuntary contractions of muscles at the base of the penis and of smooth muscles of the urethra.

Emission of semen is controlled by sympathetic nerves. Neurotransmission in these nerve terminals stimulates alpha-adrenoreceptors. This initiates contraction of seminal vesicles and the vas deferens and triggers contraction of the bulbar muscles resulting in ejaculation of semen from the urethra. Ejaculation is generally a reflex response to the entry of semen into the urethra.

Orgasm generally accompanies ejaculation, but actually precedes it by several seconds (Kollberg *et al.*, 1962). Orgasm can also occur in the absence of genital input by stimulating the septal area of the brain in humans (Heath, 1964). Orgasm has also been noted in conjunction with temporal lobe epileptic discharge (Blumer, 1970). Conceivably, some drugs may be able to produce orgasm-like sensation because of stimulation of these areas of the brain.

In the female, orgasm is associated with involuntary contractions of muscles in the perineum and surrounding areas.

4. Resolution. This is associated with decreased local vasocongestion. In the male, this is accompanied by a refractory period during which excitation cannot occur. The length of this refractory period varies among men. In the female there is no refractory phase and as a result multiple orgasms can occur in a short period of time.

SEXUAL DYSFUNCTION

Male sexual dysfunction generally involves either problems of erectile impotence or ejaculation. Erectile impotence refers to an inability to achieve or maintain an erection. Such dysfunction may arise from psychic problems which prevent sexual arousal. Psychogenic factors including fear, anxiety, or guilt are considered to be the overwhelming reasons for impotence. Impotence can also arise from physical problems such as impaired blood flow to the penis as sometimes occurs in connection with smoking.

The most common male sexual problem is premature ejaculation. This can be due to personal problems such as anxiety or local physiological factors. Premature ejaculation is more likely to occur as arousal increases. Such arousal can take the form of increased sexual excitement or anxiety and is mediated by peripheral sympathetic activation.

A third male problem is retarded ejaculation or painful ejaculation. This problem sometimes occurs in connection with heavy alcohol consumption or narcotics use, or in conjunction with drugs that affect adrenergic transmission. Antidepressants, for example, cause dry emission, retrograde ejaculation, and loss of orgasm.

Female sexual dysfunction generally involves inhibition of sexual arousal (often called frigidity), orgasmic dysfunction, or vaginismus. Inhibition of sexual desire may be due to various psychological problems that may be amenable to psychotherapy or various drugs that reduce anxiety. Physiologically, inhibition of sexual desire is accompanied by decreased vasocongestion so that vaginal lubrication may not occur.

In orgasmic dysfunction, sexual arousal may occur but never to the point of complete orgasm. This is usually associated with psychological rather than physiological factors. In contrast to the male, wherein anxiety results in premature ejaculation, in the female, anxiety is associated with delayed orgasm.

Vaginismus refers to involuntary constriction of the outer part of the vagina. Constriction can be so severe that penile entry is prevented. This may be due to psychological factors, e.g., guilt, anxiety, or physical factors, e.g., pain, stimulation of muscles.

A fourth common problem occurring in women is dyspareunia—pain associated with sexual intercourse.

Menstrual disorders are generally associated with disturbances in ovarian function. Assessment of spontaneous ovarian function is made through measurement of hormonal status—cyclic ovarian activity being controlled by the hypothalamic-pituitary-ovarian axis. Ovarian estrogen is primarily responsible for regulating this axis.

The oocytes in the ovary cause estrogen release. Ovarian dysfunction results in decreased estrogen production and increased follicle stimulating hormone (FSH) and luteinizing hormone (LH) release from the pituitary. Decreased estrogen or increased FSH/LH blood levels may thus indicate ovarian dysfunction. Amenorrhea refers to an absence of menstruation and is due to ovulatory failure. Oligomenorrhea refers to menstruation which still occurs but occurs infrequently. Anovular menstruation refers to a condition in which ovulation does not occur but cyclic uterine bleeding still takes place.

In the normal course of ovulation, there is a pulsatile rather than a gradual pre-ovulatory release of LH. If the hypothalamic area responsible for luteinizing hormone-releasing hormone (LH-RH) is affected, estrogen, FSH levels, and LH levels may be normal, but ovulation may still not occur. Decreased LH or FSH levels may indicate hypothalamic or pituitary dysfunction.

MECHANISMS OF ACTION

In affecting sexuality, drugs can act either in the brain or on peripheral nerves. Drugs which affect the brain and presumably sex centers will cause an increase or decrease in sexual arousal. Drugs that affect peripheral nerves will not affect arousal but may affect sexual function. In some cases, drug action is direct and involves chemical alteration of the neurons which underlie sexual arousal or function. Alternately, some drugs may act indirectly by altering blood flow to the genitalia.

Most hypotheses concerning the neurochemical basis of sexual behavior are derived from studies in animals, but in some cases support has come from clinical studies. The most widely endorsed of these hypotheses suggests that both serotonin and dopamine are involved in the neurochemical control of sexual behavior with serotonin playing an inhibitory role and dopamine an excitatory role. For example, drugs such as levodopa, which increase levels of dopamine in the brain, tend to be associated with increased libido and enhanced sexual function in patients suffering from abnormal dopamine activity such as that associated with Parkinsonian disease. In contrast, drugs which block dopamine function such as haloperidol cause loss of sexual arousal. There is also evidence that peptide hormones such as LHRH not only affect sexual arousal and function via their effects on endocrine systems but can also affect sexuality directly (Benkert, 1980).

Decreased sexual function is associated with drugs which inhibit adrenergic and cholinergic receptor activity such as antipsychotics like chlorpromazine (Thorazine) and thioridazine (Mellaril). These effects may be central or peripheral in origin.

RESEARCH CONSIDERATIONS

Measuring Sexual Response

Two general approaches to the question of a drug's effects on human sexual response have been taken. The first and older approach has involved indirect studies of this association through surveys and projective tests. The second and more recent approach has involved direct studies of sexual function.

Indirect Studies

(a) *Survey Studies.* The relationship between drugs and sex has been examined in a number of survey studies. Typically, a questionnaire is given to a group of people and their answers to various items are tabulated.

Such studies are of limited scientific value because they are biased in respondents, e.g., those who choose to respond, they are very subjective, e.g., definition of sexual enjoyment, and they give little or no consideration to levels of consumption.

(b) *Projective Tests.* Another indirect method of assessing a drug's effects on sexuality is through projective tests—tests that involve responses to ambiguous figures. These responses are scored for sexual imagery or content, and the tests are often administered after subjects have consumed drugs. Such studies are subject to numerous criticisms, e.g., test reliability, lack of standardization of test conditions, absence of reliable information concerning drug consumption. Especially difficult to evaluate is the significance of sexually related comments to actual behavior or sexual function.

Direct Studies

Until only recently there were no controlled studies of a drug's effects on human sexuality. During the latter half of the 1970's, however, several reports began to be published of alcohol's effects on elicited sexual arousal in men and women. These studies used the penile strain gauge to measure penile erection and the photoplethysmograph to measure vaginal blood volume and pressure. With the development of these measurement techniques, it became possible to study sexual function directly and reliably, and to correlate such changes with levels of drug use.

In his review of "Pharmacosexology," Buffum (1982) offered guidelines and procedures for conducting studies in this area. In most cases, many of the test guidelines are difficult or impossible to implement but nevertheless should be kept in mind in evaluating studies pertaining to drug effects on sexuality. These are:

1. Wherever possible, a control group should be included along with the experimental group. Since individuals have different degrees of sexual dysfunction prior to taking drugs, any changes in sexuality may be related to pre-existing conditions. For example, hypertensives tend to experience a higher incidence of sexual dysfunction even when not receiving medication than do other patients.

2. Age and marital status should be specified. Since sexuality changes with age and marital status, such information should be noted for comparison purposes.

3. The gender of the subjects should be noted. Without knowing the number of men and women studied, determining the incidence of a particular dysfunction is not feasible.

4. Use of other drugs should be noted since changes in sexuality may be due to drugs other than those being directly studied or to interactions with such drugs.

5. The method of obtaining drug-related information, e.g., systematic interview, spontaneous reporting by patients, is an important consideration. Buffum (1982) cites a number of studies showing that the incidence of a particular effect varied with the conditions under which the information was obtained.

6. Dosages of drugs should be specified.

7. Terms should be defined as clearly as possible. For example, terms such as "impotence" are ambiguous.

8. Duration of drug use should be noted. In some cases, e.g., antidepressants, drug effects do not manifest themselves for several weeks after drug use has begun. Sexual changes may also not begin until some time after drug use and may be only temporary.

9. The type of research design is critical. The best procedure involves a "double blind" assessment where neither the provider nor the user knows whether an active substance or a placebo is being administered. This minimizes "placebo effects." Randomization of patients also decreases bias as do "crossover designs" where the same individuals are assessed under drug and placebo conditions. While these conditions are often impossible to implement in sex-related studies, the more such procedures can be implemented, the more reliable the data.

References

Benkert, O. Pharmacotherapy of sexual impotence in the male. *Modern Problems in Pharmacopsychiatry*, 1980, *15*, 158–173.

Blumer, D. Hypersexual episodes in temporal lobe epilepsy. *American Journal of Psychiatry*, 1970, *126*, 8–15.

Bragonier, J. R. Influences of oral contraception on sexual response. *Medical Aspects of Human Sexuality*. 1976, *10*, 130–143.

Buffum, J. Pharmacosexology: The effects of drugs on sexual function. *Journal of Psychoactive Drugs*, 1982, *14*, 5–44.

Carney A., Bancroft, J., and Matthews, A. Combination of hormonal and psychological treatment for female sexual unresponsiveness; a comparative study. *British Journal of Psychiatry*, 1978, *133*, 339.

Freedman, A. M. Drugs and sexual behavior. Sadock, B. J., Kaplan, H. I., and Freedman, A. M. (eds.), *The Sexual experience*, Williams & Williams, Baltimore, 1976, 328–334.

Gawin, F. H. Drugs and Eros. Reflections on aphrodisiacs. *Journal of Psychedelic drugs*, 1978, *10*, 227–236.

Gay, G. R., and Sheppard, C. W. Sex in the drug culture. *Medical Aspects of Human Sexuality*, 1972, *6*, 28–47.

Heath, R. E. (ed.). *The Role of Pleasure in Behavior.* Harper and Row, New York, 1964.

Kollberg, S., Petersen, I., and Stener, I. Preliminary results of an electromyographic study of ejaculation. *Acta Chirurgia Scandinavica*, 1962, *123*, 478–482.

Kuhn, R. A. Functional capacity of the isolated human spinal cord. *Brain*, 1950, *73*, 1–51.

Masters, W. H. and Johnson, V. E. *Human Sexual Response.* Churchill, London, 1966.

Maclean, P. D. Brain mechanisms of elemental sexual functions. Sadock, B. J., Kaplan, H. I. and Freedman (eds.) *The Sexual Experience*, Williams & Williams, Baltimore, 1976, pp. 42–63.

Maclean, P. D. and Ploog, D. W. Cerebral representation of penile erection. *Journal of Neurophysiology*, 1962, *25*, 29–55.

Murray, M. A. F., Bancroft, J. H. A., Anderson, D. C., Tennent, T. G., and Carr, P. J. Endocrine changes in male sexual deviants after treatment with anti-androgens, oestrogens, or tranquilizers. *Journal of Endocrinology*, 1975, *67*, 179–188.

Chapter 1

Alcohol

Alcohol is one of the most common and most widely used substances in the world and is generally consumed in the form of beer,
wine, or distilled spirits. In small amounts it is a euphoriant. In
large amounts it causes increasing depression and loss of coordina-
tion. If consumption is excessive, it can cause loss of consciousness
and eventually death.

Alcohol is absorbed from the gastrointestinal tract, mostly
from the intestine. The more concentrated the source, the faster
the absorption. Hence the alcohol in distilled spirits, which contain
about 40 percent alcohol, is absorbed much faster than that in beer
which contains about 6 percent alcohol.

Alcohol is evenly distributed throughout all body fluids in
equal concentrations. About 95 percent of it is metabolized in the
liver and is eventually broken down into carbon dioxide and water.
The rate of metabolism is relatively slow with about one ounce of
whiskey being metabolized per hour. If more than an ounce is
consumed per hour, alcohol accumulates in the blood and various
organs.

Alcohol is a general neuronal depressant. Its euphoriant properties are presumed to result from depression of inhibitory neurons
prior to depression of excitatory neurons, resulting in "disinhibi-

tion." At higher amounts, excitatory neurons are depressed along with inhibitory neurons resulting in general depression.

Alcohol affects cell membranes, all neurochemical systems, and all endocrine systems. Consequently, it is difficult to say with any certainty that any effect is due to its actions on any specific mechanism.

MALE SEXUALITY

Throughout history men and women have searched for ways to increase or improve sexual urges, sexual performance, or sexual satisfaction, sometimes without the awareness of the other sex partner. The link between alcohol and sex seems especially timeless, as alcohol appears destined to occupy a leading place in man's arsenal of alleged aphrodisiacs for many centuries to come.

Anecdotal/Literary Evidence

For the most part, however, the association between alcohol and libido or sexual performance is highly speculative and contradictory. For example, Aristotle commented that the "semen of drunkards [is] usually infertile" (*Problemata*, 871ª23) and that "those who are drunk are incapable of having sexual intercourse" (*Problemata*, 872ª15). Alexander the Great, wrote Plutarch, often drank so much that he was "cold in love" (*Symposiacs*, 1.6). Athenaeus recorded a similar anecdote about the great conqueror: "Alexander carried his carousing to such a point . . . that he had no appetite for sexual indulgence . . ." (*Deipnosophistae*, X.435).

Plutarch also observed that "the great drinkers are very dull, inactive fellows, no women's men at all; they eject nothing strong, vigorous, and fit for generation, but are weak and unperforming, by reason of the bad digestion and coldness of their seed" (*Symposiacs*, 3.5).

Other writers, such as the twelfth-century Jewish physician-philosopher Maimonides, wrote positively concerning alcohol's effect on sexual function:

> Drinking honey water promotes erections, but even more effective in
> this regard than all medicines and foods is wine. . . .
>
> (Quoted by Benedik, 1972)

Several centuries earlier, St. Fulgentius (6th century A.D.) observed that "Venus [will] grow cold without Ceres and Bacchus" (*Mythologies*, "Of Venus"), and that "there are four stages of intoxication—that is, first, excess of wine; second, forgetting things; third, lust; fourth, madness . . ." (*Mythologies*, Dionysus). During the sixteenth century, beer was extolled for much the same reason:

> Beer brewed from wheat, above all as a beverage increases the natural
> seed, straightens the drooping phallus up again, and helps feeble men
> who are incapable of conjugal acts back into the saddle.
>
> (Quoted by Benedik, 1972)

Some writers, however, were rather circumspect about alcohol's effects and observed—to use modern pharmacological terminology—that alcohol's actions on sexual function were dose-dependent. For instance, in the fifth century B.C., the Greek poet Euenas wrote:

> The best measure of wine is neither much nor very little;
> For 'tis the cause of either grief or madness.
> Then too, 'tis most suited for the bridal chamber and love.
> And if it breathe too fiercely, it puts the Love to flight.
> And plunges men in a sleep, neighbor to death.
>
> (Quoted by Seltman, 1980)

Macrobius makes a similar observation (*Saturnalia*, 7.6):

> . . . all hot substances provoke to venery, stir the seed and favor
> procreation, but after copious draughts of unmixed wine men become
> less active lovers and the seed which they sow is unfitted for genera-
> tion, since the excess of wine, as a cold substance, makes it thin or
> weak.

Likewise, Ovid wrote that wine incited the feelings to lust, but when taken in large amounts so that one is drenched in alcohol, the senses became stupefied. Francois Rabelais, the French physician and author, similarly commented:

> . . . from intemperance, proceeding from the excessive drinking of
> strong liquor, there is brought upon the body . . . a chillness in the
> blood, a slackening in the sinews, a dissipation of the generative seed,

> a numbness and dulling of the senses, with a pervasive wryness and
> convulsion of the muscles, all of which are great lets and impediments
> to the act of generation. Wine, nevertheless, taken moderately, work-
> eth quite contrary effects. . . .
>
> (Quoted by Benedik, 1972)

The most often quoted statement about alcohol and sex is still Shakespeare's observation: "It (alcohol) provokes and unprovokes; it provokes the desire, but it takes away from the performance" (*Macbeth*, Act 2, Scene 2).

While there is a definite folklore about alcohol and sex that spans the centuries, these various examples indicate that there is also a difference of opinion in how alcohol affects sexuality.

One reason for the variety of opinions concerning alcohol and sex is due to the lack of objective information concerning this association. Until only recently, most of the information available on alcohol and sex was derived from opinions, anecdotes, and dubious questionnaires and studies. Within the last few years, however, alcohol's effects on human sexual response have begun to be studied under controlled laboratory conditions. For the most part, these studies have been conducted on men, with very little attention being devoted to alcohol's effects on female sexuality. This bias will be apparent in the following surveys of alcohol and sex in males and females. Since most of the relevant research concerns male sexuality, this information will be presented first.

Male Libido and Sexual Performance

In recent years an increasing number of studies have been conducted with respect to alcohol and male sexuality. These studies have concerned not only alcohol's acute effects on libido, penile tumescence, and ejaculatory capability, but also long-term effects on these aspects of sexual functions. In addition, considerable attention has been devoted to the effects of long-term consumption of alcohol on spermatogenesis and possible deleterious effects on offspring sired by chronic alcohol users.

Alcohol and Male Sexual Response

Two general approaches to the question of alcohol's effects on male sexual response have been taken. The first and older approach has involved indirect studies of this association through surveys and projective tests. The second and more recent approach has involved direct studies of male sexual function in response to alcohol.

Indirect Studies

(a) *Survey Studies.* The relationship between alcohol and sex has been examined in a number of survey studies. In response to a *Psychology Today* questionnaire (1970), 45% of the male respondents said alcohol increased sexual enjoyment, 42% said it decreased it, and 13% said it had no effect.

Tamerin and co-workers (1970) surveyed a small group of male alcoholics (N=13) for their beliefs concerning alcohol and sex. Most felt that intoxication decreased libido. However, during actual intoxication, most reported an increase in sexual arousal.

In a survey of patients at the Haight-Ashbury Free Medical Clinic (Gay *et al.*, 1977), of the 95 patients interviewed 46 stated that alcohol would be the last of a number of drugs (e.g., barbiturates, heroin, marihuana) that they would choose "to make sex better."

Such studies, of course, are of limited scientific value because they are biased in respondents (e.g., those who choose to respond to magazine questionnaires are very subjective (e.g., definition of sexual enjoyment), and give little or no consideration to levels of consumption.

(b) *Projective Tests.* In an early study of this type (Clark, 1952), male college students viewed a series of nude female pictures and immediately afterwards they were given the Thematic Apperception Test (TAT). A second group was given the TAT after viewing slides of landscapes. No alcohol was administered in these two conditions. The second part of this study involved TAT testing in a fraternity beer party setting where one group of men viewed nude female slides while another did not view any slides previous to being given the TAT. In the nonalcohol condition, men exposed to the nude females expressed less sexual imagery than those viewing landscapes. In the alcohol condition, the reverse was true—males exposed to the nude pictures expressed more sexual imagery. Similar results were reported by Kalin and his coworkers (1965).

In two more recent studies using the TAT projective test method, alcohol consumption did not significantly affect sexual imagery, nor were sexual responses correlated with physiological measures of sexual arousal (Briddell & Wilson, 1976; Wilson & Lawson, 1976). Later studies were conducted under more rigorous test conditions and with greater standardization. Inter-rater reliability was also higher than in the previous studies.

In summary, however, survey studies and projective test studies of alcohol and sex have generally been methodologically poor and contradictory.

Direct Studies

Until only recently there were no controlled studies of alcohol's effects on human sexuality. During the latter half of the 1970's, however, several reports began to be published of alcohol's effects on elicited sexual arousal in men and women. These studies used the penile strain gauge to measure penile erection and the photoplethysmograph to measure vaginal blood volume and pressure. With the development of these measurement techniques, it became possible to study sexual arousal directly and reliably, and to correlate such changes with levels of alcohol consumption.

The basic procedure for these studies involves administering alcohol to subjects and then showing them erotic films. Breathalyzer readings are taken before or during testing to determine blood alcohol levels.

The first such study to employ these techniques was reported by Farkas and Rosen (1976). Sixteen male college students consumed mixtures of vodka and orange juice until their blood alcohol levels reached a predetermined criterion of 0, 25, 50, or 75 mg%. Each subject acted as his own control, and order of testing was counterbalanced. After reaching criterion, the penile strain gauge was fitted and subjects reclined on a couch and watched an erotic film. Maximal tumescence, latency for tumescence, and heart rate were measured and the relationship between these responses and blood alcohol levels was determined.

Alcohol had a biphasic effect on maximal tumescence. At blood alcohol levels of 25 mg%, tumescence was increased slightly, whereas at 50 and 75 mg%, maximal tumescence was decreased. Latency for tumescence increased in a dose-related manner, as did heart rate.

This study is noteworthy for several reasons. First, it was the first to measure alcohol's effects on sexual arousal directly. Second, it correlated sexual arousal with blood alcohol levels so that it was possible to assess the relationship between alcohol and sexual arousal objectively. Third, the use of subjects as their own controls eliminated intersubject differences in experience, set, etc. Since subjects did not know what criterion blood alcohol level they were being brought to, preconceptions concerning anticipated effects of various doses were minimized.

Several additional parameters relating alcohol to sexual arousal have also been examined using this general procedure.

Rubin and Henson (1976) reported a decrease in maximal erection and increased latency to erection at blood alcohol levels of 106 mg% and above when subjects were instructed to relax. To examine the influence of "set," subjects were instructed to become aroused (in the absence of sexual stimulation). Maximal tumescence was reduced and latency to tumescence was increased at blood alcohol levels above 100 mg%, whereas below this blood alcohol level, erectile capacity was not affected. Thus, despite efforts to the contrary (attempted arousal), individuals were unable to overcome the pharmacological effects of alcohol on physiological arousal once blood alcohol levels reached 100 mg% (Wilson, 1977). However, erectile capacity was not totally suppressed at these blood alcohol levels.

Wilson and Lawson (1976) examined the effects of expectancy in conjunction with low blood alcohol levels (30–40 mg%). Half the subjects were led to believe they were drinking alcohol, whereas the other half believed they were drinking only tonic. Each of these two main groups was subdivided such that half in each group actually received alcohol or tonic in accord with their expectations. Those who believed they had consumed alcohol, regardless of whether they actually had or not, were more aroused in response to erotic films. Thus, at low blood alcohol levels, expectation, not the pharmacological effects of alcohol, is responsible for any increases in sexual arousal to erotic stimuli (Farkas & Rosen, 1976; Briddell *et al.*, 1978).

Relatively few studies have investigated the effects of alcohol on orgasmic-ejaculatory response. Survey studies (see Table 1) indicate that alcohol can cause both erectile impotence and ejaculatory incompetence. For some men, ejaculatory competence may be more affected by alcohol than erectile capacity (Powell *et al.*, 1974).

A direct study of alcohol's influence on ejaculatory competence was recently reported by Malatesta *et al.* (1979). Twenty-four nonalcoholic males were tested in five sessions. Subjects served as their own controls. During the first session, subjects were "desensitized." In the next four sessions, subjects were given alcohol to bring their blood alcohol levels to 0, 30, 60, or 90 mg%. They were then shown erotic films and were instructed to masturbate until reaching orgasm and ejaculation. Latency of ejaculation was determined by measuring genital muscle activity and by direct subject response. Ejaculatory latency was increased with increasing blood alcohol levels. Ten of the twenty-four subjects were unable to achieve ejaculation at the highest blood alcohol level.

Studies of alcohol's effects on erectile capacity and ejaculatory competence have also been conducted with animals (Gantt, 1952; Tietelbaum & Gantt, 1958). In these studies, penile arousal in dogs was produced manually and occurrence of erection, latency of erection, and ejaculation were determined under alcohol and non-alcohol conditions. Although the levels of alcohol studied were much greater than those used to study human male sexual response, these early experiments likewise demonstrated a dose-related inhibition of sexual arousal by alcohol. The use of animals, of course, precludes confounding of factors such as "expectations," "set," "setting," etc.

Clinical Studies

Chronic alcoholism has been associated with sexual dysfunction in several studies (see Table 1). In Lemere and Smith's study (1973) of 17,000 alcoholics, 8% suffered from erectile impotence. Even after several years of sobriety, one-half of this group of 8% remained impotent, although they still expressed an interest in sex.

Other studies, with the exception of Powell *et al.* (1974), report an even higher incidence of erectile impotence among alcoholics (See Table 1). Whalley (1978), confirmed the incidence of erectile impotence among alcoholics. Compared to a 54% incidence among alcoholics, the incidence among non-alcoholics matched for age and social class was 28%.

Although consistent with experimental studies of alcohol's effects on sexual arousal, these clinical studies leave unanswered the issue of pharmacological versus psychological factors. For exam-

TABLE 1. Incidence (%) of Sexual Dysfunction among Alcoholics

Reference	Erectile impotence	Premature ejaculation	Ejaculatory incompetence
Akhtar (1977)			
(N = 45)	31.1	6.6	17.8
Lemere and Smith (1973)			
(N = 17,000)	8		
Powell *et al.* (1974)			
Alcoholics	4 sober, 24 drunk		0 sober, 18 drunk
Nonalcoholics	0 sober, 10 drunk		0 sober, 28 drunk
Whalley (1978)			
(50 per group)			
Alcoholics	54		
Nonalcoholics	28		

ple, impotence could be due to guilt feelings associated with sex, and alcohol may initially be a means of dealing with these underlying guilt feelings. For example, Ewing (1968) reported that alcohol improved the problem of premature ejaculation in 23 patients (out of 200). However, the amount of alcohol consumed had to be carefully monitored because excessive consumption resulted in delayed ejaculation or impotence (Viamontes, 1974). Thus, depending on dosage, alcohol may improve sexual performance when "psychological" factors underlie sexual dysfunction. Nevertheless, consumption of alcohol may also be a primary causal factor in impotence due to its pharmacological actions on the mechanisms underlying erectile capacity (see below).

EFFECTS ON HORMONES

Chronic alcohol abuse in man frequently results in feminization and hypogonadism. Feminization is often associated with liver dysfunction (Lloyd & Williams, 1948), resulting in increased clearance of testosterone and decreased clearance of estrogens. The latter may be due to resorption of estrogens into the blood due to liver disease (Van Thiel *et al.*, 1979). To the extent that male libido is affected by the balance between male and female sex steroid levels, alcohol-related effects on such steroids will affect male libido whether alcohol acts directly on the testes or indirectly on mechanisms related to testes function.

At present, the reduction in testosterone levels associated with alcohol ingestion appears to be due to a dual effect of alcohol on both the Leydig cells and on the hypothalamic-pituitary-gonadal axis (HPG axis) (Cicero *et al.*, 1979; Van Thiel *et al.*, 1974a).

Direct evidence that alcohol inhibits Leydig cell function comes from *in vitro* studies in which testosterone production by Leydig cells is first stimulated by chorionic gonadotropin or cyclic AMP after which the experiment is repeated in the presence of alcohol in concentrations comparable to those generally encountered during intoxication. In one such study (Ellingboe & Varanelli, 1979), alcohol produced a dose-related reduction in testosterone production beginning at 10 mg%. Similar results were reported by Cobb and his co-workers (1978).

The primary site for alcohol's effects on the HPG axis appears to be the hypothalamus. This conclusion is based on the observation that alcohol does not affect the release of LH from the pituitary by LH-RH, e.g., Symons & Marks, 1975; Leppaluoto *et al.*, 1975; Cicero *et al.*, 1978.

Additional evidence that alcohol acts on the HPG axis is derived from the fact that levels of LH tend to be within normal limits in alcoholics (Gordon *et al.*, 1976; Lester & Van Thiel, 1977; Van Thiel *et al.*, 1974b) instead of being elevated, as would be expected as a result of the negative feedback relationship between the components of the HPG axis. The absence of a compensatory increase in LH levels when testosterone production is decreased by alcohol (Cicero, 1980) suggests alcohol impairment of the HPG axis (Cicero, 1980).

In addition to the effects of alcohol on Leydig cell function and the HPG axis, alcohol also appears to lower testosterone levels by increasing the rate by which the liver metabolizes this hormone (Gordon *et al.*, 1976, 1975, 1976, 1978; Rubin *et al.*, 1976).

Thus, chronic alcohol ingestion in man and animals can result in lower serum testosterone levels through a number of different biological mechanisms. In contrast to the effects of chronic alcohol ingestion, however, studies of the effects of acute exposure to alcohol have not produced consistent results (Leppaluoto *et al.*, 1975; Gordon *et al.*, 1976; Mendelson *et al.*, 1977; Ylikahri *et al.*, 1978.) This inconsistency may be due to methodological factors. For instance, depending on dosage and time of sampling after administration, alcohol is capable of producing different results (Cicero & Badger, 1978).

NEURAL FACTORS

The fact that alcohol-related impotence often occurs in the absence of decreased libido (Teitelbaum & Gantt, 1958) suggests that neurological damage to the reflex mechanisms involved has occurred. Furthermore, studies of paraplegic animals and men indicate that alcohol can inhibit erectile and ejaculatory processes due to its direct actions on the spinal neurons underlying these reflexes.

For example, priapism in paraplegic men is inhibited following subarachnoid injection of alcohol into their lumbar area (Sheldon & Bors, 1948). Similarly, in dogs and rats with midthoracic spinal transsection, alcohol will inhibit erectile and ejaculatory reflexes normally produced by penile stimulation (Hart, 1968; 1969).

While penile erectile and ejaculatory competence is inhibited at the reflex level by alcohol, this does not necessarily mean that the "higher" cortical centers underlying sex are unaffected by alcohol. However, these studies are consistent with experimental data (see above) indicating that despite attempted arousal, individuals are unable to overcome the pharmacological effects of alcohol above certain blood alcohol levels.

Effects on Sperm

In addition to loss of libido and impaired sexual performance, chronic alcohol consumption produces hypogonadism and eventual sterility. It is also possible that sperm production may be adversely affected to the point at which conception of defective offspring could occur. Plato (*Laws*, 6.775–776), for instance, cautioned that "when drunk, a man is clumsy and bad at sowing seed, and is thus likely to beget unstable and untrusty offspring, crooked in form and character." Similarly, in Roman mythology, the deformed god Vulcan was said to have been conceived while his father Jupiter was drunk. Whether the Greeks and Romans actually appreciated the possibility that alcohol could adversely affect sperm production is uncertain since these anecdotes might have simply reflected a plea for moderation in general.

Modern recognition of alcohol's link with gonadal dysfunction in men can be traced back to the early nineteenth century (Arlit & Wells, 1917). Gonadal dysfunction is frequently associated with liver disease, but also occurs in connection with alcoholism when liver disease is mild or absent (Arlit & Wells, 1917; Anderson *et al.* 1980; Klassen & Persaud, 1978). One important characteristic of such dysfunction is sperm damage and eventual aspermia.

Initially, alcohol interferes with production of spermatozoa from spermatids. As a result of the reduced conversion of spermatids to spermatozoa, the seminiferous tubules fill with spermatids. The spermatids eventually degenerate and disappear from the tubules as well. Ultimately, spermatocyte and spermatogonia production are inhibited and complete aspermia occurs. In this regard it is interesting to note that in rape cases, sperm has not been found in vaginal secretions when the rapist is an alcoholic.

Alcohol-induced sterility may also result from alcohol-related scarring of the vas deferens. The scarring produced by alcohol not only obstructs the vas deferens, but also subsequently results in testicular atrophy, decreases in seminiferous tubule diameter, and Leydig cell damage (Dixit *et al.*, 1976; Freeman, 1975; Freeman, 1973; Raman *et al.*, 1976).

Yet another mechanism whereby alcohol may produce sterility is the inhibition of testicular conversion of retinol (Vitamin A) to retinal by alcohol dehydrogenase. Retinol is essential for spermatogenesis. When ingested, retinol is oxidized to retinal by alcohol dehydrogenase. By competing with retinol for ADH, alcohol reduces retinal production. Although sustained levels of blood alcohol would be required to reduce retinal levels to the point that spermatogenesis would be affected, such sustained levels are not out of the realm of possibility, as suggested by the increased incidence of "night blindness" in alcoholics (Van Thiel *et al.*, 1974), also related to competitive inhibition of retinal.

Alcohol is not only capable of inhibiting spermatogenesis, it may also reduce sperm motility and increase the incidence of morphological abnormalities in sperm prior to the occurrence of aspermia (Van Thiel & Lester, 1976). The spermatozoa produced often lack normal tails.

The concentration of alcohol in sperm is almost identical to that in blood (Doepfmer & Hinckers, 1965), and following ingestion of alcohol, sperm motility is significantly decreased (Doepfmer & Hinckers, 1965; Beck & Hinckers, 1972; Farrell, 1938; Sharma & Chaudhury, 1970).

Abnormalities in sperm morphology have been observed in male alcoholics who are able to produce an ejaculate. Among the anomalies noted are double-headed spermatozoa, irregularly arranged mitochondria, absence of acrosomes, anomalies in the acrosome, malformations of the nucleus, broken off heads, curled tails, and distended midsections (Lester & Van Thiel, 1977; Semczuk, 1978).

Although not all sperms produced by male alcoholics are damaged, there is the possibility that damaged sperms could fertilize an ovum. There are few definite data at present, however, indicating that alcoholic men can sire children who are adversely affected by such a parentage. Nevertheless, considerable indirect evidence points to such a possibility.

PATERNAL FACTORS IN FETAL ALCOHOL EFFECTS

Whereas no significant increases in the frequency of anomalies have been noted among offspring of male alcoholics or male animals that consumed alcohol, experiments in animals suggest that paternal alcohol consumption is capable of producing other kinds of damage to the developing fetus.

Among early studies, Nice (1917) reported lower birth weights in offspring of mice sired by males given alcohol. Nice also noted an increase in postnatal mortality among offspring of sires given alcohol. Stockard and Papanicolaou (1916, 1918), reported a fivefold increase in the stillbirth rate of progeny sired by male guinea pigs given alcohol. Compared to a postnatal mortality rate of 19/118 for controls, the stillbirth rate for offspring of alcohol-treated males was 35/82.

More recent studies on litter size of animals sired by males that consumed alcohol are summarized in Table 2.

Badr and Badr (1975) reported that average litter size de-

TABLE 2. Litter Size in Offspring Sired by Alcohol-Consuming Males
($\bar{x}$ ± S.E.)

Species	Alcohol	Control	Reference
Mouse	4.4 (±0.8)	7.2 (±0.5)	Badr & Badr (1975)
Mouse	4 (±1)	8 (±2)	Anderson *et al.* (1978)
Rat	7.0 (±2.5)	12.1 (±0.5%)	Klassen & Persaud (1976)

creased when female mice were mated with males that had received alcohol (0.1 ml, 40% v/v, p.o.) for only three days. In this
study, males were placed with a different group of females every
fourth day and the effect on litter size was noted when matings
occurred 14–17 days after alcohol exposure.

Klassen and Persaud (1976) likewise observed a decrease in
litter size in offspring sired by males consuming alcohol. In this
study, male rats consumed liquid alcohol diets for 15 to 35 days.
Control rats were given an isocaloric diet but were not pair-fed so
that while it is unlikely, the observed effects could have been due
to nutritional factors. In addition to decreased litter size, resorption
rate was increased considerably in litters sired by alcohol-consuming males, whereas fetal weight and length were both reduced.

Although no details were given, Pfeifer and co-workers (1977)
reported decreased litter size and increased postnatal mortality in
offspring sired by alcohol-consuming male rats. The authors also
reported behavioral anomalies in these offspring but again no details were given.

Anderson and co-workers (1978) placed male mice that had
previously sired at least one litter on a liquid alcohol diet (5% v/v)
for 26 days. Two days after males ceased consuming alcohol, they
were bred. Exposure to alcohol did not affect conception rate, but
litter size was significantly smaller and postnatal mortality was
significantly increased among offspring sired by alcohol-consuming males.

The decreased litter sizes observed in dams mated with alcohol-consuming males could have been the result of decreased

sperm motility, impaired ability of sperm to fertilize ova, damage to sperm resulting in dominant lethal mutations, or transmission of nongenetic material from sperm to ova which resulted in lethal mutations.

Although decreased sperm motility has been noted among male alcoholics (see above), no such evidence was observed in male mice given alcohol (Anderson *et al.* 1978), nor is there evidence of decreased fertility on the part of alcohol-consuming male animals (Anderson *et al.*, 1980; 1978). There is also no evidence that alcohol produces chromosomal damage in sperm.

In summary, animal studies suggest that male alcohol consumption has the potential for increasing pre- and postnatal mortality of sired offspring. The mechanisms for this effect are unknown as yet. Whether a comparable effect occurs in humans is also unknown.

SUMMARY AND CONCLUSIONS

In summary, consumption of relatively moderate amounts of alcohol can result in increased sexual arousal. However, this "aphrodisiac" effect is due to expectations, not to any pharmacological action. At blood alcohol levels of 50 mg% or more (approximately 3 "drinks") pharmacological effects begin to manifest themselves and sexual arousal (as indicated by tumescence) does not occur as readily as with lower blood alcohol levels. At blood alcohol levels of 100 mg% or more, sexual arousal (i.e., tumescence) is significantly inhibited and ejaculatory competence is eliminated in many men. Although these conclusions are based on nonalcoholic male college students, similar results have also been observed in chronic alcoholics tested under similar conditions (Lemere & Smith, 1973) as well as in animals.

The loss of libido commonly encountered in male alcoholics is likely due to decreased testosterone levels. At least three different mechanisms have been identified whereby such decreases may occur. Cortical centers integrating and regulating the motivational basis of sex (i.e., libido) could conceivably be affected wither directly by alcohol or indirectly through decreased testosterone levels. However, in the case of alcohol-related effects on testosterone levels, it should be noted that (a) testosterone levels are lowered, not eliminated; and (b) while male libido is affected by sex steroids, these do not act as "motivators" but rather as "primers" for responding to certain kinds of stimuli. Reduction in testosterone levels thus might dampen libido, but such a reduction would not necessarily suppress libido completely.

In conclusion, the evidence from a number of different sources is consistent in showing that alcohol does not stimulate libido in men. Any suggestion to the contrary is the result of expectancies in the absence of pharmacological actions of alcohol. As consumption of alcohol increases, the pharmacological actions of alcohol express themselves despite expectations and instead of an increase in libido and sexual potency, libido is decreased and erectile and ejaculatory competence are reduced. These changes in libido and potency are the result of both an overall depression in physiological function and specific effects on male sex steroid production and neural reflex mechanisms.

FEMALE SEXUALITY

One of the most pervasive "double standards" in history associated with sex involves alcohol. Whereas men have praised alcohol as an elixir vitae for weary libidos, they have at the same time carefully regulated the alcohol consumption of their wives and daughters for feat that drinking might lead to promiscuity.

Anecdotal/Literary Evidence

The early Romans were very circumspect in their use of wine and during the times of the kings of Rome women were not even permitted to drink it. Pliny (*Natural History* 14.90) says that some women were even put to death by their husbands if caught drinking! Athenaeus (*Dipnosophistae* X.440) also refers to such as law as do other Roman writers. The law apparently ceased to be enforced around the second century B.C. (*Dipnosophistae*, X.440).

Behind this law was the belief that wine was a powerful aphrodisiac for women rather than the perception of any ill effects on offspring. Dionysius of Halicarnassus (*Roman Antiquities* 2.25.6) wrote that Romulus considered drinking by women and adultery to be similar crimes. Polybius (*History*, 6.2) wrote that "it is almost impossible for them (women) to drink wine without being found out. For the woman does not have charge of the wine; moreover, she is bound to kiss all of her male relatives and those of her husband down to her second cousins every day on seeing them for the first time; and as she cannot tell which of them she will meet she has to be on her guard."

Dionysius of Halicarnassus (1st century B.C.) attributes an ancient law against allowing women to drink to Rome's founder, Romulus. Women guilty of wine-drinking could be punished with death since, according to Romulus, drunkenness was the source of adultery.

The rabbis of Talmudic times were especially cautious about giving wine to women because of its potential as a sexual inciter:

> One glass of wine is becoming to a woman, two are somewhat degrading, and if she has three glasses she solicits coitus, but if she has four, she solicits even an ass in the streets and forgets all decency.
>
> (*Ketuboth*, 65a)

Clement of Alexandria also cautioned women about their drinking:

> As for women, who are especially trained in good manners, if only they would not keep their lips wide open as they drink from big cups, with their mouths distorted out of shape. And if only they would not lean their heads back when they drain vessels narrow of neck, thereby exposing their throats with—or so it seems to me—such immodesty. They hold their chins high as they pour the drink down, as if they were trying to reveal as much of themselves as they can to their companions at table . . . and their carousals begin to play the coquette. . . . A woman is quickly drawn into immorality even by only giving consent to pleasure.
>
> (*Christ the Educator*, 2.2)

Basil (4th century A.D.) wrote a homily "Against Drunkeness" directly as a result of a scene he witnessed during Easter Sunday when some girls entered a church in Antioch and began drinking, dancing, and singing indecent songs, and urged many of the men around to join them, which they did. Basil describes many of the physical and cognitive effects of drunkenness, among which he says, men lose all inhibitions where sex is concerned and behave like animals (*Homilies*, 14.3) and women act like common harlots (*Homilies*, 14.8).

In the Canons of the Holy Apostles, written about the 4th century A.D., the faithful were warned not to drink to the point of drunkenness and the evils of such drinking are ennumerated (Book 8, no. 44) indicating that such problems were commonplace and were of concern to the Church Fathers.

Chrysostom (4th century A.D.) condemned the drunkenness he saw all around him and also ennumerated the adverse consequences in his sermons of drinking to excess. Chrysostom also worried about the many women who became drunk (Gospel of St. Matthew, Homily 57, 5.6). In one Homily (24) he again writes about the firmly held belief in alcohol's aphrodisiac effects: "For from banquets of that sort you have evil desires, and impurities, and harlots in honor among you. . . . Wherefore I beseech you flee fornication, and the mother of it, drunkenness."

Ambrose, Bishop of Milan (4th century A.D.), dutifully listed the many effects of drunkeness on the body and behavior and said that drinking and adultery were so closely connected that one did not occur without the other (*De Viduis,* 7.40).

To Jerome (4th century A.D.) the greatest sin associated with drunkenness was sexual licentiousness: "Venus shivers unless Ceres and Bacchus be with her" (*Adversus Jovinianum* 2.7). Wine heats the body, said Jerome, and the heat boils over into lust (Epistles 69.9). Both girls and monks should drink water, Jerome advised, so that the natural heat of their bodies would be cooled (Epistles 54.10).

Bishop Fulgentius (6th century A.D.) carries the same thought into the next century and wrote in "The Fable of Dionysus" that:

"There are four stages of intoxication—that is, first, excess of wine; second, forgetting things; third, lust; fourth madness—whereby these four received the name of Bacchae" (*Mythologies*, 12).

Many centuries later, in *The Canterbury Tales* (the prologue to "The Wife of Bath's Tale"), Geoffrey Chaucer has the Wife of Bath confess what others only hinted:

> After wine, I think mostly of Venus
> For just as it's true that cold engenders hail
> A liquorous mouth must have a liquorous tail.
> Women have no defense against wine
> As lechers know from experience.

The notion that alcohol has the potential to arouse promiscuity in women is still heard in ditties or light verse such as Ogden Nash's "Candy is dandy,/But liquor is quicker."

Alcohol, as these anecdotes imply, has been regarded throughout history as an aphrodisiac where women are concerned and as a weapon for unscrupulous men to lull otherwise provident women into sexual abandon.

In general, relatively little information exists concerning alcohol's effects on female sexuality beyond these anecdotes. Carpenter and Armenti's remark that "most experts comment on human sexual behavior and alcohol as though only males drink and have sexual interests" (p. 521) is as relevant today as a decade ago. In the last few years, however, some epidemiological and experimental studies regarding alcohol and female libido and sexual function have begun to appear. Although there is still much more to be learned concerning alcohol and female sexuality, the taboo surrounding this general area of study seems to be less rigidly enforced and many more studies of this association will undoubtedly be appearing in the near future.

Indirect Studies

Survey Studies. In the *Psychology Today* study (1970) of alcohol and human sexuality discussed in the previous chapter, women were also asked to respond to the questionnaire. Of those who did respond, 68% felt alcohol increased sexual enjoyment, 21% reported a decrease, and 11% stated it had no effect.

In the Gay *et al.* survey (1977) of women (N=36) from San Francisco's Haight-Ashbury district, most reported alcohol played a minor role in sexual enhancement.

The many criticisms mentioned previously in connection with such studies (see above) make it difficult to attach much significance to these results.

In a more recent and much better controlled study, Beckman (1979) surveyed alcoholic women and nonalcoholic control women concerning their behavior and feelings regarding sex after drinking. A third group of women in treatment for psychiatric or emotional disorders was also surveyed. Nonalcoholic controls were matched with alcoholics in age, marital status, education, religion, and parity.

The data comparing alcoholic and nonalcoholic women are shown in Table 3. More alcoholic women stated that they desired intercourse most when drinking, more enjoyed sex most when drinking, and more alcoholic women said they actually engaged in sex most when drinking. Women with psychiatric or emotional problems were more like control women than alcoholic women in their feelings and sexual behavior when drinking.

Several studies characterize female alcoholics as sexually unre-

TABLE 3. Desire for, Enjoyment of, and Engagement in Sexual Intercourse While Drinking or Not Drinking among Alcoholic (A) and Nonalcoholic (NA) Women[a]

	% Desiring sex most		% Enjoying sex most		% Engaging in sex most	
	A	NA	A	NA	A	NA
When drinking	57	29	55	32	55	25
When not drinking	20	19	30	23	21	25
No difference	24	51	16	45	23	50

[a]Table adapted from Beckman (1979).

sponsive or dissatisfied, but sexually "promiscuous" (Curran, 1937; Kinsey, 1968; Levine, 1955; Schuckit, 1972; Wood & Duffy, 1966; Wall, 1937; Myerson, 1959; Lisansky, 1957). Myerson (1959) comments that "their promiscuity during their drinking episodes is sometimes so chaotic and involves so many men that there is no way of knowing who sired the resultant child."

Promiscuity, however, defies objective definition. No matter how it is defined, it may be less characteristic of female alcoholism than of particular subgroups (Schuckit, 1972; Lisansky, 1957).

Paradoxically, female alcoholics tend to be childless more often than nonalcoholics, and have larger families than non-alcoholics (Mowrer & Mowrer, 1945; Rosenbaum, 1958; Wilsnack, 1973). This paradox may be due, on the one hand, to greater infertility on the part of some alcoholics, and due, on the other hand, to a greater need in those alcoholics who are fertile to prove their femininity by the size of their families.

Thus, alcohol is associated with increased sexuality for many women, especially "alcoholics." However, this does not necessarily mean that alcohol has "aphrodisiac" properties nor does it mean that alcohol increases sexual responsiveness. For women who are insecure about their sex role identities, increased sexuality may be one way to reassure themselves of their femininity. As in the case of men, women associate alcohol with sex. Depending on the availability of sex partners, the setting, and opportunities for sexual liaison, alcohol may simply be a means for many women to "act out" desired sex roles.

Direct Studies

The development of the vaginal photoplethysmograph, a device for measuring vaginal blood volume and pressure, has permitted objective studies of female sexual responsiveness. The general method for studying alcohol's effects on sexual arousal in women using this device is similar to studies in men using the penile strain gauge (see above). Women consume varying amounts of alcohol, they view or listen to erotic material, their breath alcohol levels and physiological responses are monitored, and they are questioned concerning their subjective feelings of arousal.

In two studies (Wilson & Lawson, 1976, 1978), blood alcohol levels of 0–79 mg% produced a dose-related decrease in physiological sexual arousal as reflected by vaginal pressure. However, in contrast to their physiological response, women reported increased feelings of sexual arousal. The results occurred regardless of expectancies (Wilson & Lawson, 1978), i.e., women who were led to believe they had not been given alcohol, but in fact had received it, did not differ significantly from those who expected and actually received alcohol. Similarly, those that believed they had been given alcohol, but had been given a placebo, did not differ from those that believed they had not been given alcohol and actually did not receive it.

A difference between objective and subjective measures of sexual arousal in women has also been reported by Malatesta and co-workers (1980). In this study, increasing blood alcohol levels (25–75 mg%) increased latency and decreased intensity of orgasmic response (produced by masturbation). In contrast to these decreases in physiological arousal, women reported a dose-related increase in subjective sexual arousal and pleasure from orgasm.

These studies in women contrast with those in men in an interesting way. In men, alcohol decreased both objective and subjective measures of sexual arousal (Malatesta *et al.*, 1979), whereas in women objective measures of arousal were decreased while subjective measures were increased.

With respect to women and drinking in general, however, these studies do not support the pervasive "disinhibition" theory whereby alcohol allegedly "releases" inhibitions normally controlling expression of sexual behavior (Block, 1965; Goodwin, 1976). As posited by this theory, sexual behavior is constantly seeking an outlet, but is held in check by inhibiting cortical mechanisms. Freed from restraint, everyone would be either a satyr or nymphomaniac.

Nor do the data support the social learning theory, whereby sexual behavior is dependent on previous reinforcements. "Although individuals appear to lose control," argues Wilson (1977), "unconventional sexual behavior seems to have occurred not in spite of, but consistent with operative reinforcement contingencies" (p. 249). In other words, sexual activity does not occur more often in the context of drinking because moral inhibitions or restraints are overcome or "disinhibited." Rather, it occurs because people act in accord with what they have learned society expects drinking to lead to. The expectation is fulfilled in accord with what has been learned. Drinking, then, becomes an excuse, if one is needed, to avoid responsibility for behavior—"I never would have done it, had I been sober."

The fact that many women feel sexually aroused by alcohol, whether they are physiologically aroused or not (Beckman, 1979; Wilson & Lawson, 1976; 1978; Malatesta *et al.*, 1980; Wilsnack, 1981), suggests that alcohol does in fact have "aphrodisiac" properties in women to a certain degree. Whether these perceived feelings are acted upon may depend on setting, availability of sex partners, and "operative reinforcement contingencies."

Clinical Studies

Gynecological problems have frequently been noted among female alcoholics. Uncertain, however, is whether these problems are the result of alcohol consumption or whether they precipitate such dysfunction. Major difficulties in resolving this issue are the absence of control groups against which to compare female alcoholics, the need to distinguish between subgroups of female alcoholics, reliance on self-report data, and absence of information concerning time relations between onset of drinking and dysfunction (Wilsnack, 1981).

MENSTRUAL DISORDERS

Menstrual disorders, e.g., dysmenorrhea, menorrhagia, appear to occur frequently among alcoholic women.

As early as 1876, Haddon remarked on how common irregular

menstrual cycles and menorrhagia seemed to be among alcoholic women.

Wall (1937) reported that 40 of the 50 alcoholic women he studied had a history of dysmenorrhea. Gynecological examination at the time of hospital residence did not reveal any pelvic pathology to account for the disorder.

Moscovic (1975) surveyed 321 chronic alcoholic women in obstetrical/gynecological clinics in Yugoslavia. Approximately two-thirds of these women had ovarian dysfunction. The most common problems were oligomenorrhea (30.8%), hypomenorrhea (18.2%), dysmenorrhea (15.6%), polymenorrhea (13.2%), and amenorrhea (10.6%). Although he could not study the time sequence of these problems, Moscovic noted that ovarian dysfunction occurred more frequently in women over 30 years of age compared to those between 20 and 25, suggesting that ovarian dysfunction occurred more often in later life for these women after alcohol had had time to produce dysfunction.

In addition to these menstrual problems, 8.7% of the alcoholics in the Moscovic study had early onset of menopause (prior to 40 years of age), which is considerably higher than the 4% rate for the general population in Yugoslavia (Moskovic, 1975).

Jones and co-workers (1980) have also noted a considerably earlier onset of menopause among alcoholic women compared to controls of the same age (average age 44 and 42 years, respectively). These observations should be investigated more thoroughly since they suggest that alcohol may have been a precipitating factor in early onset of menopause. If menopause had precipitated alcoholism, the alcohol problem would not have developed until the late forties or fifties.

Beckman (1979) reported that 51% of a group of alcoholic women had "menstrual or other female problems" compared to 36% for controls. However, among a group of psychiatric-treatment women, the incidence of these problems was 54%. This similarity in incidence of dysfunction between alcoholic and psychiatric patient populations suggests that alcohol is not the sole factor responsible for menstrual problems among alcoholics.

Again, while they have not discerned the sequence of drinking and gynecological problems, several authors have reported that many alcoholic women drink more heavily during premenstruum, and many attribute their drinking to the desire to relieve menstrual distress (Beckman, 1979; Belfer *et al.*, 1971; James, 1975; Lolli, 1953; Podolsky, 1963). Conceivably, endocrine imbalances may be one of the factors precipitating alcoholism for some women who are already heavy drinkers (Baird, 1979). However, the obverse is also plausible, viz., heavy drinking may precipitate hormonal imbalances leading to premenstrual distress.

Effects on Hormones

Menstrual disorders are generally associated with disturbances in ovarian function (Baird, 1979). Assessment of spontaneous ovarian function is made through measurement of hormonal status—cyclic ovarian activity being controlled by the hypothalamic-pituitary-ovarian axis. Ovarian estrogen is primarily responsible for regulating this axis.

The oocytes in the ovary cause estrogen release. Ovarian dysfunction results in decreased estrogen production and increased follicle stimulating hormone (FSH) and luteinizing hormone (LH) release from the pituitary. Decreased estrogen or increased FSH/LH blood levels may thus indicate ovarian dysfunction.

There are few studies of alcohol's effects on hormonal levels in women. Acute alcohol consumption resulting in blood alcohol levels of 118 mg% did not affect serum LH, FSH, progesterone, or prolactin levels in nonalcoholic women (N=8). Women in this study were tested during the follicular phase of their menstrual cycles and blood samples were drawn at various times after alcohol ingestion (McNamee *et al.*, 1979).

LH, FSH, and prolactin levels also did not differ in postmenopausal alcoholic women compared to nonalcoholic controls, nor did these alcoholic women differ in their elevated LH and FSH responses to LH–RH administration (Hugues & co-workers, 1978).

In animal studies, administration of 2, 3, or 8 g/kg/day of alcohol for 12 consecutive days also did not affect plasma LH levels in rats, although normal estrous cycles were disrupted (Eskay & coworkers, 1981). Blake (1974; 1974) reported that alcohol did not affect pituitary release of LH in response to LH–RH in rats, suggesting that alcohol does not affect pituitary sensitivity to LH–RH.

Alcohol has been reported to block ovulation in various species of animals including rabbits (Saul, 1959), rats (Kieffer & Ketchel, 1970), and mice (Cranston, 1958). In some cases, this effect has been attributed to alcohol's direct actions on the ovary.

Van Thiel and co-workers (1978) reported that the ovaries of female rats consuming a liquid alcohol diet (5% v/v) for 7 weeks weighed two-fifths that of pair-fed controls. The uterus and fallopian tubes of alcohol-fed animals weighed about one-fourth that of controls. Ovarian examination revealed an absence of large, well-developed follicles, corpus lutea, and corpus hemorrhagia in alcohol-fed rats. Histological examination showed that the endometrium and fallopian tubes in the alcohol-fed animals contained only a single layer of secretory cells suggestive of estrogen deprivation. Plasma LH and FSH levels in alcohol-treated animals did not differ from pair-fed controls, but plasma estradiol levels were significantly reduced.

Reductions in uterine weights and alterations in morphology of the uterus, ovaries, and vagina in rats following ingestion of alcohol for about 50 days has also been reported by Bo and co-workers (1981).

These studies suggest that alcohol can affect ovarian function directly as a gonadal toxin and possibly indirectly by affecting hypothalamic release of hormones necessary for ovulation.

Infertility in female animals has also been produced by administration of alcohol into the uterus. However, in most cases the concentration of alcohol used has been very high. For example, Conner and co-workers (1976) injected pregnant rats on gestation days 3 or 7 with alcohol (50–100% v/v). Injections were made directly into the uterus through the cervix. Dams were sacrificed on gestation day 15. When injected on gestation day 3, nearly all embryos were dead (*cf.* Brent, 1978).

Zipper and co-workers (1968) injected alcohol (50 or 100% v/v) directly into one of the uterine horns of nonpregnant rats and then placed them with males. Rates of implantation were normal in the untreated uterine horn, but sterility was observed in the treated horn. In some cases, sterility was reversed by the fourth month after treatment.

Dubin and his co-workers (1978) demonstrated that alcohol could terminate pregnancy in monkeys even when locally applied to the amniotic sac. The alcohol (70% v/v) was applied extra-amniotically through the cervix by a blunt needle. All monkeys resumed menstrual cycles within a year of treatment but only three became pregnant.

Alcohol has also been used to induce mid-term abortion in women (Gomel & Carpenter, 1973). Amniotic fluid was first removed and then replaced by a comparable volume of fluid containing alcohol (47.5%). Fetal heart sounds disappeared within an hour after alcohol administration. Abortions occurred spontaneously between 20 hours and 40 days after treatment. The final concentration of alcohol in the amniotic fluid was estimated at between 100 and 150 mg%.

Spontaneous Abortion

Alcoholic women tend to be both childless more often and to have larger families than nonalcoholics. Increased family size has been attributed to the need, on the part of the alcoholic woman, to prove her femininity (Wilsnack, 1981). The reasons for the increased incidence of childless families among alcoholics, however, may be due to alcohol's effects on the reproductive system. Since women who drink heavily also tend to be married to men who are heavy drinkers (Gomberg, 1975), and since alcohol adversely affects sperm production, childlessness among alcoholic women may be due to male aspermia or to male-induced dominant lethal mutations as well.

There is evidence, however, that alcohol is in fact related to sterility in women. Wilsnack (1973) for example, found that alcoholic women had greater difficulty in conceiving and in carrying pregnancies to term compared to other married women matched for age, socioeconomic status, and ethnicity.

Harlap and Shiono (1980) have also reported a dose-related increase in the number of spontaneous abortions associated with alcohol consumption. With consumption of one drink per day, the risk factor for spontaneous abortion during the first trimester was 1.12. With three or more drinks, the risk factor increased to 1.16. However, during the second trimester, the risk factor increased from 1.03 for one drink per day to 3.53 for consumption of 3 or more drinks per day.

Kline and her co-workers (1980) have also reported an increase in spontaneous abortions associated with alcohol. The threshold for increasing the risk of spontaneous abortion was two drinks, consumed twice weekly, with wine conveying the highest risk.

SUMMARY AND CONCLUSIONS

Although a great deal has been written about the effects of alcohol on female sexuality and reproductive function, there is very little objective information concerning these subjects. Much of what has previously been claimed is based on speculation, or studies of men. Whereas there are now a few studies of alcohol's effects on female sexuality and reproductive function, the reliability of these studies must remain tentative until corroborated or refuted by other studies. Nevertheless, based on the available information, a number of generalizations are now possible.

The first generalization is that, as in the case of alcoholism and problem drinking in general, the effects of alcohol on female sexuality and reproductive function must be considered separately from male sexuality and reproduction. This generalization goes beyond the obvious male-female differences in hormonal cycles. Male subjective responsiveness to alcohol mirrors physiological response as far as sex is concerned, whereas in females this does not necessarily occur. Alcohol may in fact have an "aphrodisiac"-like effect in women that is not observed in men.

The second generalization is that excessive alcohol consumption adversely affects ovarian function. This results in various menstrual disorders and infertility.

The third generalization is that alcohol consumption significantly increases the risk of spontaneous abortion, particularly during the second trimester of pregnancy.

Studies in animals clearly demonstrate that alcohol is capable of adversely affecting female reproductive function and fecundity. One apparent site of action for these effects is the ovary itself. It is also possible that hypothalamic sites that monitor the levels of circulating sex hormones and release the hormone(s) that regulate pituitary function are also adversely affected by alcohol. Studies in animals also have shown that alcohol can induce abortion; indeed, alcohol has been used clinically for that purpose.

References

Akhtar, J. J. Sexual Disorders in Male Alcoholics. *Alcoholism and drug dependence: A multidisciplinary approach.* J. S. Madden, R. Walker and W. H. Kenyon (Eds.), Plenum Press, New York, 1977, 3–12.

Anderson, R. A., Beyler, S. A. and Zaneveld, L. J. D. Alterations of male reproduction induced by chronic ingestion of ethanol: Development of an animal model. *Fertility and Sterility,* 1978, *30,* 103–105.

Anderson, R. A., Willis, B. R., Oswald, C., Reddy, J. M., Beyler, S. A. and Zaneveld, L. J. D. Hormonal imbalance and alterations in testicular morphology induced by chronic ingestion of ethanol. *Biochemical Pharmacology,* 1980, *29,* 1409–1419.

Arlit, A. H. and Wells, H. G. The Effect of Alcohol on the Reproductive Tissues. *Journal of Experimental Medicine,* 1917, *26,* 769–782.

Badr, F. M. and Badr, R. S. Induction of dominant lethal mutation in male mice by ethyl alcohol. *Nature,* 1975, *253,* 134–136.

Baird, D. T. Endocrinology of Female Infertility. *British Medical Bulletin,* 1979, *35,* 193–198.

Beck, K. J. and Hinckers, H. J. Untersuchungen uber den Ubertritt von Alkohol in den Zervikalmukus und seine Bedeutung fur die Sterilitat der Frau. *Geburtshilfe und Frauenheilkunde,* 1972, *32,* 585–589.

Beckman, L. J. Reported effects of alcohol on the sexual feelings and behavior of women alcoholics and nonalcoholics. *Journal of Studies on Alcohol,* 1979, *40,* 272–282.

Belfer, M. L., Shader, R. I., Carroll, M., and Harmatz, J. S. Alcoholism in Women. *Archives of General Psychiatry,* 1971, *25,* 540–544.

Benedik, T. G. Food and drink as aphrodisiacs. *Sexual Behavior,* 1972, *2,* 5–10.

Blake, C. A. Centrally acting drugs must inhibit spontaneous neural stimulation of luteinizing hormone release for a specific 7-hour period to block ovulation in rats. *Federation Proceedings: Federation of American Societies for Experimental Biology,* 1974, *33 Part 1,* 221.

Blake, C. A. Differentiation between the "Critical Period", the "Activation Period" and the "Potential Activation Period" for neurohumoral stimulation of LH release in proestrous rats. *Endocrinology,* 1974, *95,* 572–578.

Block, M. A. *Alcoholism: Its facets and phases.* John Day, New York, 1965.

Bo, W. J., Krueger, W. A., Rudeen, P. K., and Symmes, S. K. The effect of different doses of ethanol on ovarian function. *Alcoholism: Clinical and Experimental Research,* 1981, *5,* 349.

Brent, R. L. Vulnerability of the preimplantation mammalian embryo. *Teratology* 1978, *17,* 17A.

Briddell, D. W. and Wilson, G. T. Effects of alcohol and expectancy set on male sexual arousal. *Journal of Abnormal Psychology,* 1976, *85,* 225–234.

Briddell, D. W., Rimm, D. C., Caddy, G. R., Krawitz, G., Sholis, D. and Wunderlin, R. J. Effects of alcohol and cognitive set on sexual arousal to deviant stimuli. *Journal of Abnormal Psychology,* 1978, *87,* 418–430.

Carpenter, J. A. and Armenti, N. P. Some effects of ethanol on human sexual and aggressive behavior. In *The biology of alcoholism* (vol. 2), *Physiology and behavior.* B. Kissin and H. Begleiter (Eds.), Plenum Press, New York, 1972, 509–543.

Cicero, T. J. and Badger, T. M. Effects of alcohol on anterior pituitary secretion of the tropic hormones. *Journal of Clinical Endocrinology & Metabolism,* 1978, *46,* 715–720.

Cicero, T. J., Bernstein, D., and Badger, T. M. Effects of acute alcohol administration on reproductive endocrinology in the male rat. *Alcoholism: Clinical and Experimental Research,* 1978, *2,* 249–254.

Cicero, T. J., Meyer, E. R., and Bell, R. D. Effects of ethanol on the hypothalamic pituitary luteinizing hormone axis and testicular steroidogenesis. *Journal of Pharmacology and Experimental Therapeutics,* 1979, *208,* 210–215.

Cicero, T. J. Sex Differences in the Effects of Alcohol and Other Psychoactive Drugs on Endocrine Function. *Alcohol and Drug Problems in Women,* D. J. Kalant (Ed.). Plenum Press, New York, 1980, 545–593.

Clark, R. A. The projective measurement of experimentally induced levels of sexual motivation. *Journal of Experimental Psychology,* 1952, *44,* 391–399.

Cobb, C. F., Ennis, M. F., Van Thiel, D. H., Gavaler, J. S., and Lester, R. Acetaldehyde and ethanol are direct testicular toxins. *Surgical Forum,* 1978, *29,* 955–958.

Conner, E. A., Blake, D. A., Parmley, T. H., Burnett, L. S., and King, T. M. Efficacy of various locally applied chemicals as contragestational agents in rats. *Contraception,* 1976, *13,* 571–582.

Cranston, E. M. Effect of tranquilizers and other agents on sexual cycle in mice. *Proceedings of the Society of Experimental Biology and Medicine,* 1958, *98,* 320–322.

Curran, F. J. Personality studies in alcoholic women. *Journal of Nervous and Mental Disease,* 1937, *86,* 645.

Dixit, V. P., Agrawal, M., and Lohiya, N. K. Effects of a single ethanol injection into the Vas Deferens on the testicular function of rats. *Endokrinologie* 1976, *67,* 8–13.

Doepfmer, R. and Hinckers, H. J. Zur Frage der Keimschadigung im Akuten Rausch. *Zeitschrift fur Haut und Geschlechtskranheiten,* 1965, *39,* 94–107.

Dubin, N. H., Blake, D. H., Parmley, T. H., Conner, E. A., Cox, R. T., and King, T. M. Intrauterine ethanol-induced termination of pregnancy in cynomolgus monkeys (*Macaca Fascicularis*). *American Journal of Obstetrics and Gynecology,* 1978, *132,* 789–790.

Ellingboe, J. and Varanelli, C. C. Ethanol inhibits testosterone biosyntheses by direct action on Leydig cells. *Research Communications in Chemical Pathology and Pharmacology,* 1979, *24,* 87–102.

Enos, W. F. and Beyer, J. C. Prostatic acid phosphatase, aspermia, and alcoholism in rape cases. *Journal of Forensic Science,* 1980, *25,* 353–356.

Eskay, R. L., Ryback, R. S., Goldman, M., and Majchrowicz, E. Effect of chronic ethanol administration on plasma levels of LH and the estrous cycle in the female rat. *Alcoholism: Clinical and Experimental Research,* 1981, *5,* 204–206.

Ewing, J. A. Alcohol, sex, and marriage. *Medical Aspects of Human Sexuality,* 1968, *4,* 43–50.

Farkas, G. M. and Rosen, R. C. Effect of alcohol on elicited male sexual response. *Journal of Studies on Alcohol,* 1976, *37,* 265–272.

Farrell, J. I. The secretion of alcohol by the genital tract: An experimental study. *Journal of Urology,* 1938, *40,* 62–65.

Freeman, C. and Coffey, D. S. Male sterility induced by ethanol injection into the Vas Deferens. *International Journal of Fertility,* 1973, *18,* 129–132.

Freeman, C. Preliminary human trial of a new male sterilization procedure: Vas Sclerosing. *Fertility and Sterility,* 1975, *26,* 162–166.

Gantt, W. H. Effect of alcohol in the sexual reflexes of normal and neurotic male dogs. *Psychosomatic Medicine,* 1952, *14,* 174–181.

Gay, G. R., Newmeyer, J. A., Elion, R. A., and Weiner, S. The sensuous hippie. Part I: drug/sex practice in the Haight-Ashbury. *Drug Forum,* 1977, *6,* 27–47.

Gomberg, E. S. Alcoholism and women: State of knowledge today. Paper presented at the National Alcoholism Forum, Milwaukee, Wisconsin, 1975.

Gomel, V. and Carpenter, C. W. Induction of midtrimester abortion with intrauterine alcohol. *Journal of Obstetrics and Gynecology,* 1973, *41,* 455–458.

Goodwin, D. *Is alcoholism hereditary?* Oxford University Press, New York, 1976.

Gordon, G. G., Olivo, J., Rafin, F., and Southren, A. L. Conversion of androgens to estrogens in cirrhosis of the liver. *Journal of Clinical Endocrinology and Metabolism,* 1975, *40,* 1018–1026.

Gordon, G. G., Altman, K., Southren, A. L., Rubin, E., and Lieber, C. S. Effect of alcohol (ethanol) administration on sex-hormone metabolism in normal men. *New England Journal of Medicine,* 1976, *295,* 793–797.

Gordon, G. G., Southren, A. L., and Lieber, C. S. The effects of alcoholic liver disease and alcohol ingestion on sex hormone levels. *Alcoholism: Clinical and Experimental Research,* 1978, *2,* 259–263.

Haddon, J. On Intemperance in Women, with Special Reference to its Effects on the Reproductive System. *British Medical Journal,* 1876, *1,* 748–750.

Harlap, S. and Shiono, P. H. Alcohol, smoking, and incidence of spontaneous abortions in the first and second trimester. *Lancet,* 1980, *2,* 173–176.

Hart, B. L. Effects of alcohol on sexual reflexes and mating behavior in the male dog. *Quarterly Journal of Studies on Alcohol*, 1968, 29, 839–844.

Hart, B. L. Effects of alcohol on sexual reflexes and mating behavior in the male rat. *Psychopharmacologia*, 1969, 14, 377–382.

Hugues, J. N., Perret, G., Adessi, G., Costs, T., and Modigliani, E. Effects of chronic alcoholism on the pituitary-gonadal function of women during menopausal transition and in the post menopausal period. *Biomedicine Express*, 1978, 29, 279–283.

James, J. E. Symptoms of alcoholism in women: A preliminary survey of A. A. members. *Journal of Studies on Alcohol*, 1975, 36, 1564–1569.

Jones, B. M., Jones, M. K., and Hatcher, E. M. Cognitive deficits in women alcoholics as a function of gynecological status. *Journal of Studies in Alcohol*, 1980, 41, 140–146.

Kalin, R., McClelland, D. C., and Kahn, M. The effects of male social drinking on fantasy. *Journal of Personality and Social Psychology*, 1965, 1, 441–452.

Kieffer, J. D. and Ketchel, M. M. Blockade of ovulation in the rat by ethanol. *Acta Endocrinologica*, 1970, 65, 117–124.

Kinsey, B. A. Psychological factors in alcoholic women from a state hospital sample. *American Journal of Psychiatry*, 1968, 124, 1463–1466.

Klassen, R. W. and Persaud, T. V. N. Experimental studies on the influence of male alcoholism on pregnancy and progeny. *Experimentelle Pathologie*, 1976, 12, 38–45.

Klassen, R. W. and Persaud, T. V. N. Influence of alcohol on the reproductive system of the male rat. *International Journal of Fertility*, 1978, 23, 176–184.

Kline, J., Shrout, P., Stein, Z., Susser, M., and Warburton, D. Drinking during pregnancy and spontaneous abortion. *Lancet*, 1980, 2, 176–180.

Kuhn, R. A. Functional capacity of the isolated human spinal cord. *Brain*, 1950, 73, 1–51.

Lemere, F. and Smith, J. W. Alcohol-induced sexual impotence. *American Journal of Psychiatry*, 1973, 130, 212–213.

Leppaluoto, J., Rapeli, M., Varis, R., and Ranta, T. Secretion of anterior pituitary hormones in man: Effect of ethyl alcohol. *Acta Physiologica Scandinavica*, 1975, 95, 400–406.

Lester, R. and Van Thiel, D. H. Gonodal Function in Chronic Alcoholism. *Advances in Experimental Medicine and Biology*, 1977, 85A, 399–414.

Levine, J. The sexual adjustment of alcoholics: A clinical study of a selected sample. *Quarterly Journal of Studies on Alcohol*, 1955, 16, 675–680.

Lisansky, E. S. Alcoholism in women: Social and psychological concomitants. Social history data. *Quarterly Journal of Studies on Alcohol*, 1957, 18, 588–623.

Lloyd, C. W. and Williams, R. H. Endocrine changes associated with Laennec's cirrhosis of the liver. *American Journal of Medicine*, 1948, 4, 315–330.

Lolli, G. Alcoholism in women. *Connecticut Review on Alcoholism*, 1953, 5, 9–11.

Malatesta, V. J., Pollack, R. H., Wilbanks, W. A., and Adams, H. E. Alcohol effects on the orgasmic-ejaculatory response in human males. *Journal of Sex Research*, 1979, 15, 101–107.

Malatesta, V. J., Pollack, R. H., Crotty, T. D., and Peacock, L. J. Acute alcohol intoxication and the female orgasmic response. *Journal of Sex Research*, 1982, *18*, 1–17.

McNamee, B., Grant, J., Ratcliffe, J., Ratcliffe, W., and Oliver, J. Lack of effect of alcohol on pituitary-gonadal hormones in women. *British Journal of Addiction*, 1979, *73*, 316–317.

Mendelson, J. H., Mello, N. K., and Ellingboe, J. Effects of acute alcohol intake on pituitary-gonadal hormones in normal human males. *Journal of Pharmacology and Experimental Therapeutics*, 1977, *202*, 676–682.

Moskovic, S. Uticaj Hronicnog Trovanja Alkoholom na Ovarijunsku Disfunkciju. *Srpski Arhiv a Celokupno Lekarstvo*, 1975, 751–758.

Mowrer, E. R. and Mowrer, H. Ecological and familial factors associated with inebrity. *Quarterly Journal of Studies on Alcohol*, 1945, *6*, 30–44.

Myerson, D. J. Clinical observations on a group of alcoholic prisoners. *Quarterly Journal of Studies on Alcohol*, 1959, 555–572.

Nice, L. B. Further observations on the effects of alcohol on white mice. *American Naturalist*, 1917, *51*, 596–607.

Pfeifer, W. D., MacKinnon, J. R., and Seiser, R. L. Adverse effects of paternal alcohol consumption of offspring in the rat. *Bulletin of the Psychonomic Society*, 1977, *10*, 246.

Podalsky, E. The woman alcoholic and premenstrual tension. *Journal of the American Medical Women's Association*, 1963, *18*, 816–818.

Powell, B. J., Viamontes, J. A., and Brown, C. S. Alcohol effects on the sexual potency of alcoholic and nonalcoholic males. *Alcoholism*, 1974, *10*, 78–80.

Psychology Today. Sex. *Psychology Today*, July 1970, 30–52.

Raman, G., Purandare, T. V., and Munshi, S. R. Sterility induced in male rats by injection of chemical agents into the Vas Deferens. *Andrologia*, 1976, *8*, 321–325.

Rosenbaum, B. Married women alcoholics at the Washingtonian hospital. *Quarterly Journal of Studies on Alcohol*, 1958, *19*, 79–89.

Rubin, H. B. and Henson, D. E. Effects of alcohol on male sexual responding. *Psychopharmacology*, 1976, *47*, 123–134.

Rubin, E., Lieber, C. S., Altman, K., Gordon, G. G., and Southren, A. L. Prolonged ethanol consumption increases testosterone metabolism in the liver. *Science*, 1976, *191*, 563–564.

Saul, G. Blockade of ovulation in the rabbit by intoxicating doses of ethyl alcohol. *Anatomical Record*, 1959, *133*, 332.

Schuckit, M. A. Sexual disturbance in the woman alcoholic. *Medical Aspects of Human Sexuality*, 1972, *6*, 44–62.

Seltman, C. *Wine in the ancient world*. Routledge and Kegan Paul, London, 1980.

Semczuk, M. Further investigations on the ultrastructure of spermatozoa in chronic alcoholics. *Zeitschrift fur Mikroskipisch—Anatomische Forschung* 1978, *92*, 494–508.

Sharma, S. C. and Chaudhury, R. R. Studies on mating. Part II: The effect of ethanol on sperm transport and ovulation in successfully mated rabbits. *Indian Journal of Medical Research*, 1970, *58*, 501–504.

Sheldon, C. H. and Bors, E. Subarachnoid alcohol block in paraplegia: Its beneficial effect on mass reflexes and bladder dysfunction. *Journal of Neurosurgery*, 1948, 5, 385–391.

Stockard, C. R. and Papanicolaou, G. A further analysis of the hereditary transmission of degeneracy and deformities in the descendants of alcoholized mammals. *American Naturalist*, 1916, 50, 65–88, 144–177.

Stockard, C. R. and Papanicolaou, G. A. Further studies on the modification of the germ cells in mammals: The effect of alcohol on treated guinea-pigs and their descendants. *Journal of Experimental Zoology*, 1918, 26, 119–226.

Symons, A. M. and Marks, V. The effects of alcohol on weight gain and the hypo-thalamic-pituitary-gonadotrophin axis in the maturing male rat. *Biochemical Pharmacology*, 1975, 24, 955–958.

Tamerin, J. S., Weiner, S., and Mendelson, J. H. Alcoholics expectancies and recall of experiences during intoxication. *American Journal of Psychiatry*, 1970, 126, 39–46.

Teitelbaum, H. A. and Gantt, W. H. The effects of alcohol on sexual reflexes and sperm count in the dog. *Quarterly Journal of Studies on Alcohol*, 1958, 19, 394–398.

Van Thiel, D. H. Feminization of Chronic Alcoholic Men: A Formulation. *Yale Journal of Biology and Medicine*, 1979, 52, 219–225.

Van Thiel, D. H., Gavaler, J. S., and Lester, R. Ethanol inhibition of vitamin A metabolism in the testes: Possible mechanism for sterility in alcoholics. *Science*, 1974, 186, 941–942.

Van Thiel, D. H., Lester, R., and Sherins, R. J. Hypogonadism in alcoholic liver disease: Evidence for a double defect. *Gastroenterology*, 1974, 67, 1188–1194.

Van Thiel, D. H. and Lester, R. Alcoholism: Its effect on hypothalamic-pituitary-gonadal function. *Gastroenterology*, 1976, 71, 318–327.

Van Thiel, D. H., Gavaler, J. S., and Lester, R. Alcohol-induced ovarian failure in the rat. *Journal of Clinical Investigation*, 1978, 61, 624–632.

Van Thiel, D. H., Gavaler, J. S., Cobb, C. F., Sherins, B. J., and Lester, R. Alcohol-induced testicular atrophy in the adult male rat. *Endocrinology*, 1979, 105, 888–895.

Viamontes, J. A. Alcohol abuse and sexual dysfunction. *Medical Aspects of Human Sexuality*, 1974, 8, 185–187.

Wall, J. H. A study of alcoholism in women. *American Journal of Psychiatry*, 1937, 93, 943.

Whalley, L. J. Sexual adjustment of male alcoholics. *Acta Psychiatrica Scandinavica*, 1978, 58, 281–298.

Wilsnack, S. C. Sex role identity in female alcoholism. *Journal of Abnormal Psychology*, 1973, 82, 253–261.

Wilsnack, S. C. Alcohol, sexuality, and reproductive dysfunction in women. *Fetal Alcohol Syndrome*. E. L. Abel (Ed.), CRC Press, Boca Raton, Florida, 1982.

Wilson, G. T. and Lawson, D. M. Expectancies, alcohol, and sexual arousal in male social drinkers. *Journal of Abnormal Psychology*, 1976, 85, 587–594.

Wilson, G. T. and Lawson, D. M. Effects of alcohol on sexual arousal in women. *Journal of Abnormal Psychology*, 1976, 85, 489–497.

Wilson, G. T. Alcohol and human sexual behavior. *Behavior Research and Therapy*, 1977, 15, 239–252.

Wilson, G. T., Lawson, D. M., and Abrams, D. B. Effects of alcohol on sexual arousal in male alcoholics. *Journal of Abnormal Psychology*, 1978, *87*, 609–616.

Wilson, G. T. and Lawson, D. M. Expectancies, alcohol, and sexual arousal in women. *Journal of Abnormal Psychology*, 1978, *87*, 358–367.

Wood, H. P. and Duffy, E. L. Psychosocial factors in alcoholic women. *American Journal of Psychiatry*, 1966, *123*, 341.

Ylikahri, R., Huttunen, M. O., Harkonen, M., Leino, T., Helenius, T., Liewendahl, K., and Karonen, S. Acute effects of alcohol on anterior pituitary secretion of the tropic hormones. *Journal of Clinical Endocrinology & Metabolism*, 1978, *46*, 715–720.

Zipper, J., Mendel, M., and Prager, R. Alterations in fertility induced by unilateral intrauterine instillation of cytotoxic compounds in rats. *American Journal of Obstetrics and Gynecology*, 1968, *101*, 971–978.

Chapter 2

Amphetamines

The amphetamines, dextroamphetamine (Dexedrine), methamphetamine (Desoxyn), and *dl*-amphetamine (Benzedrine), are potent CNS stimulants. First synthesized in the 1930s to relieve nasal congestion, Benzedrine's stimulant properties were quickly recognized and during World War II they were widely used in the armed forces to increase alertness.

Amphetamines are taken orally or intravenously, although usually methamphetamine is the only amphetamine to be taken the latter way. When used sporadically and in low doses (60 mg or less), amphetamines produce mood elevation and increased alertness, hence their designation as "uppers." When used in higher doses and chronically, they produce a number of physical disorders, such as rapid heart rate, high blood pressure, and irregular heart beat, which can be life threatening. Other life threatening effects include hyperthermia. Psychologically, excessive use is associated with "amphetamine psychosis," a condition similar to paranoid schizophrenia.

Chronic use of amphetamines can result in tolerance to many of their CNS effects resulting in use of higher doses and development of physical dependence. Withdrawal is characterized by irritability, sleep disturbances, fatigue, and emotional depression.

The primary sites of action for these drugs in the brain are the reticular activating system and the cortex. Their mechanism of action involves mimicry of the adrenergic neurotransmitters, norepinephrine and dopamine. This occurs as a result of direct stimulation of adrenergic receptors, inhibition of norepinephrine reuptake into nerve endings thereby prolonging its actions, and as a result of inhibition of monoamine oxidase, the enzyme which metabolizes norepinephrine.

MDA (3,4-methylene-dioxyamphetamine) is a derivative of amphetamine which has received some attention in terms of its effects on sexuality. This drug is generally taken orally and produces euphoria and relaxation. Specific effects are discussed below.

As noted by Smith and his co-workers (1978), "belief in the aphrodisiacal effect of amphetamine pervades both the drug culture and general statements made by investigators about the relation of drugs to sexual function. This appears to be a general property of central nervous system (CNS) stimulants" (p. 228). Despite the pervasiveness of this belief, Dahlberg (1971) comments that "heavy prolonged amphetamine use can serve to prevent orgasm in the male without impairing the ability to have an erection. Later, complete impotence ensues. Less certain are the effects of prolonged high-dose amphetamine use on the female, but there is some reason to think that menstrual disorders and frigidity can result" (p. 71).

These differences in opinion are reflected by clinical studies which report that amphetamine use is associated with increased libido and sexuality in some patients, decreased effects in others, and no effects on libido or sexual functions in still others. Studies and reports addressing these different conclusions are examined below.

Literary/Anecdotal Reports

In contrast to drugs such as alcohol, morphine, heroin, and cocaine, there are considerably fewer literary and anecdotal reports concerning amphetamine's effects on sex.

In general, the immediate effects of intravenously administered amphetamine are often compared to sexual orgasm and are termed a "rush" or "flash." In their discussion of this reaction, Carey and Mandell (1968) quote one respondent's experience as follows: "When it's done right, when the needle goes into your arm, it hurts, but it's like a sexual excitement—when the speed goes into your veins, you flash out—that's sort of like a shock. Then, you get the rush, which is accompanied by a feeling of euphoria" (p. 167).

Parr (1976) quotes some amphetamine users in his study as regarding these drugs as "the greatest aphrodisiac" which produces "fantastic sex." However, other users commented that "speed destroys desire and capacity." Among the reported effects on sexual function were prolonged erection, delayed ejaculation, and multiple orgasms in both men and women.

Angrist and Gershon (1969) also comment on reports by amphetamine users they studied to the effect that the drug produced "marathon" sexual relations consisting of increased libido and delayed ejaculation.

Most of the anecdotal comments about amphetamines and their effects on sex are of this nature, with their emphasis on enhanced libido and sexual performance. Noteworthy is the fact that such reports nearly always refer to intravaneous administration of the drug.

MALE SEXUALITY

Case Studies

Information from clinical reports can be cited to support all possible effects of amphetamines on libido and sexual function. For example, shortly after its widespread introduction into clinical use, several clinicians commented that their patients experienced increased libido after using amphetamines (e.g., Bett, 1946; Carr, 1954; Hampton, 1961; Korns and Randell, 1938; Monroe and Drell, 1947; Norman and Shea, 1945; Waud, 1938; Schilder, 1938).

Reports based on larger patient populations corroborate the impression that the effects of amphetamines on libido and sexual functions are highly unreliable. Connell (1958) reported that 7 out of the 17 amphetamine users he studied reported increased libido following amphetamine use, five experienced a decrease, and five experienced no effect on libido. Bell and Trethowan (1961) noted that among their 14 amphetamine-using patients, five experienced increased sexuality, three experienced decreased sexuality, and five did not experience any change in sexuality. (Not enough information was available for the remaining patient.) Among those patients reporting increased sexuality, the effects were delayed ejaculation, resulting in prolonged sexual intercourse. Decreased sexuality took the form of depressed libido and performance.

Angrist and Gershon's (1969) findings are similar. Although none of their amphetamine users appear to have experienced decreased sexuality, only 8 out of 43 reported an enhancement of sexual function.

Several studies have also been conducted in which volunteers in drug rehabilitation or treatment centers were surveyed as to amphetamine's effects on their libido and sexual function.

In an early study reported by Nail and co-workers (1974), increased sexuality was not cited as the reason for amphetamine use by men in the navy who had volunteered for drug rehabilitation, although this was the main reason given for cocaine use.

Shiorring (1977) interviewed 50 Scandinavian amphetamine users who were in treatment for their drug problem. Eighty-five percent claimed that they experienced "strong" sexual stimulation after taking amphetamines.

In the first of three studies reported by Gay and Sheppard (1973), thirty of the thirty-six "speed freaks" interviewed at the Haight Ashbury Free Medical Clinic claimed that their sexual drive was increased by amphetamines, especially after intravenous use. Of the eighteen men who had used amphetamines intravenously, ten claimed that the drug caused immediate erection, whereas three out of the eighteen female users claimed injection produced immediate orgasm. Multiple orgasms were also reported by ten out of the eighteen males and five out of the eighteen female users. However, five of the eighteen men and three of the women reported inability to achieve orgasm after amphetamine use.

Gay and Sheppard (1973) comment that the amphetamine-induced orgasm resulting from intravenous use "is the motivating factor for use in many cases, with shared sexual activity a secondary factor." In either case, a desire for sexual activity is almost always reported (p. 34).

In a second study, Gay and his co-workers (1977) surveyed another group of drug users. For those who used amphetamines for sexual reasons, the preferred route of administration was by injection. Among the group as a whole, however, amphetamines were not cited as affecting sexuality to any major extent, but amphetamines were chosen second in response to the question "what drug would you choose over having sex with anyone of your choice?"

In a third study, Gay *et al.* (1982) reported that heterosexual, bisexual, and homosexual women all rated amphetamines as the drug they would be least likely to use "to make sex better." Males did not reject amphetamines to the same extent as women, and they did not endorse amphetamines for sexual enhancement. Amphetamines were also rarely cited as increasing sexual pleasure.

As is apparent from these latter three studies, the regard for amphetamines as sexual enhancers has decreased considerably. This decreased regard may be due to the new perceived status of other drugs, e.g., cocaine, amyl nitrites, or disenchantment with the concomitant effects of its chronic amphetamine use, or both.

These reports underscore the variability in the reaction to amphetamines as far as sex is concerned. The clinical studies are especially difficult to evaluate since the clinical populations studied were generally characterized by pre-existing psychopathologies involving sexual and social adjustment. Also worth noting is the fact that the amphetamine dosages to which these patients were exposed varied from 50 to 100 mg per day, and patients differed in their frequency of usage.

Despite the many problems inherent in these studies, some attempts have been made to account for the differences in responsiveness to amphetamines. Bell and Trethowan (1961) suggested that amphetamines have little effect on libido or sexual activity when the user's pre-existing problem is "inhibited sexuality." Both Bell and Trethowan (1961) and Angrist and Gershon (1969) comment that while amphetamines may increase sex drive, sexuality tends to be regressive in terms of increased masturbation and homosexuality. Schick *et al.* (1972) relate this regressiveness as possibly due to amphetamine-related increases in impulsive behavior similar to the stereotyped behavior of animals given amphetamines. Some observations tend to support this theory. For example, in their study of adolescents in England, Scott and Willcox (1965) noted that "in three cases parents complained that their sons had, on returning home in amphetamine intoxication, openly masturbated. 'He sat down in front of the television, opened his trousers and started playing with himself. His sister was in the room; he didn't seem to know we were there" (p. 873). Angrist and Gershon (1976) comment that "increased promiscuity, compulsive masturbation, prostitution, and intensification of sadomasochistic fantasies were all reported as consistent sequelae of amphetamine use" (in their patients). In a later study reported by Angrist and Gershon (1976) in which they administered amphetamine to nine chronic amphetamine users, they reported that "one subject experienced increased sexual tension and compulsive masturbation each time he received amphetamine." A second subject "became guilty and preoccupied with past homosexual experiences and complained that "another patient had made homosexual advances toward him" (denied by the other patient). A third subject, "the one female subject in the group became seductive and then propositioned the investigator during the study."

Smith and co-workers (1978) have called attention to the fact that despite the relative lack of specific information concerning amphetamine use and sex, generalizations have nevertheless been made about this relationship. These generalizations, they note, are often biased by researchers' value judgments. For example, some of the researchers whose work they cite have regarded homosexuality and group sex as perversions or deviance, which Smith *et al.* (1978) contend, does not reflect current thinking by many others in the field of human sexuality. As a result of these biases, generalizations such as amphetamine-induced "regression," "promiscuity," and "perversion" (e.g., Bell & Trethowan, 1961; Angrist & Gershon, 1969) must be reappraised.

SEXUAL BEHAVIOR IN ANIMALS

Crowley and co-workers (1974) reported that while methamphetamine increased activity, decreased food-seeking behavior, and affected dominance-submissive roles in a colony of monkeys, it did not affect sexual behaviors.

In contrast to this observation, Schiorring (1977) reported that amphetamine did affect sexual behavior in monkeys. In this study, a stable sexual pattern developed during a 3 month non-drug period between a male and two females such that one of the females was preferred but the male eventually mounted both. After amphetamine treatments, the male either masturbated (which never occurred during placebo treatment), or switched his sexual interest to only one of the females.

Lowe (1938) reported that although cocaine was ineffective in increasing terminal ejaculation volume before death in mice, benzedrine did produce a small but significant increase in ejaculation volume.

Soulairac (1963) observed a biphasic effect of amphetamine on sexual behavior in male rats. At a dose of 2mg/kg (i.p.), ejaculatory frequency was initially increased and the post ejaculatory refractory period was decreased. However, with continued administration opposite effects were noted. No details were reported as to whether females were sexually receptive, or if males had had previous sexual experience, both of which could have affected the outcome of this study.

Bignami (1966) also observed increased sexual activity in male rats treated with a low dose of amphetamine (0.5 mg/kg). At doses of 2 mg/kg, intromission frequency was decreased.

Leavitt's (1969) studies in this area are the most thorough and best designed. In his studies, male rats with previous sexual experience were tested in a familiar environment with females in estrus. Sexual behavior was generally increased by the two amphetamine doses studied (0.75 mg/kg and 2.25 mg/kg). The latency decrease for intromission (time between introduction of female and first successful intromission) was statistically significant. General motor activity was significantly increased by both doses.

MENSTRUATION

Although there are some reports of altered menstrual function associated with use of amphetamines, e.g., increased duration and cramping, these reports are inconsistent (Stoffer *et al.*, 1969) and will require considerably more information before any evaluation can be attempted.

MDA

Although MDA (3,4-methylene-dioxy-amphetamine) has a "street" reputation as the "love drug," or "speed for lovers," there is little specific information concerning its effects on sex. Weil (1976) relates that MDA decreases the desire for orgasm. Several reports also call attention to enhanced interpersonal relations characterized as "love" which may evoke sexual activity (Jackson & Reed, 1970); Gay and Sheppard (1973) report that 15 of their 20 respondents claimed that MDA produced "erotic fantasies" and a "compelling 'speedlike sex drive'." Three users reported prolonged intercourse and multiple orgasms.

In their second study (Gay *et al.*, 1977), MDA was noted as being cited highly among drugs used "to make sex better." However, it was rated second overall among drugs that increased sexual pleasure. Among lesbian women, MDA was rated as highest in this latter category and was rated second highest among bisexual women.

SUMMARY AND CONCLUSIONS

Amphetamine use is associated with increased libido and delayed ejaculation for a number of users. This effect occurs in a small proportion of users and mostly among those who take amphetamines intravenously. In part, this may be due to the act of injection per se, rather than effects of the drug.

On the basis of their extensive interviews and surveys with amphetamine users, Smith and co-workers (1978) have drawn the following conclusions with respect to amphetamine's effects on libido and sexual performance. Low doses, taken orally, are associated with enhanced libido and euphoria. Sustained erections and delayed ejaculation often occur at low doses—an effect considered positive in nature for men. Women also reported increased libido and prolonged pelvic thrusting at low doses, but there is less agreement about their ability to achieve orgasm. At moderate doses, increasing sexual dysfunction occurs among both men and women. For men, this takes the form of inability to achieve erection and orgasm; in women, higher amphetamine dosage also prevents orgasm (although for some men and women, multiple orgasms are experienced). At high doses, particularly when route of administration is intravenous, a "pharmacogenic orgasm" occurs for some users which acts as a substitute for sex. In some cases, where both men and women were injecting the drug, sexual activity may be replaced by mutual amphetamine injection. In still other instances, sexual activity that deviates from an individual's normal sexual behavior may emerge, such as group sex, marathon sex, or homosexual sex. In addition, men may experience impotence and women may experience an inability to achieve orgasm. As in the case of most psychoactive drugs, the effects of amphetamines on sex can vary in the same person depending on dose, route of administration, drug tolerance, "set," and "setting." In general, episodic use is more often associated with sexual enhancement than is habitual use. In the case of sustained and prolonged intravenous use (a "run") libido and sexual activity are greatest during the beginning of the run with loss of sexual interest occurring as usage continued. The latter may be a secondary result of exhaustion. For some individuals, one component of the increase in libido is associated with injection per se. This reaction has also been noted in conjunction with narcotics users who inject their drugs intravenously. Although there are relatively few studies in animals evaluating the effects on sexual activity, in general, the relevant literature is in agreement with these conclusions.

References

Angrist, B. and Gershon, S. Clinical effects of amphetamine and L-dopa on sexuality and agression. *Comprehensive Psychiatry*, 1976, *17*, 715–722.

Angrist, B. M. and Gershon, S. Amphetamine abuse in New York City—1966 to 1968. *Seminars in Psychiatry*, 1969, *1*, 195–207.

Bell, D. S. and Trethowan, W. H. Amphetamine addiction and disturbed sexuality. *Archives of General Psychiatry*, 1961, *4*, 74–78.

Bett, W. R. Benzedrine sulfate in clinical medicine: A survey for the literature. *Post Graduate Medical Journal*, 1946, *22*, 205–222.

Bignami, G. Pharmacological influences on mating behavior in the male rat. *Psychopharmacology*, 1966, *10*, 44–58.

Carey, J. T. and Mandell, J. A San Francisco bay area "speed" scene. *Journal of Health & Social Behavior*, 1968, *9*, 164–174.

Carr, R. B. Acute psychotic reaction after inhaling methamphetamine. *British Medical Journal*, 1954, *1*, 1476–1483.

Connell, P. Amphetamine psychosis. *Institute of Psychiatry Maudsley Monographs No. 5*, 1958, 51–52.

Crowley, .T. J., Stynes, A. J., Hydinger, M., and Kaufman, I. C. Ethanon, Methamphetamine, Pentobarbital, Morphine, and Monkey Social Behavior. *Archives of General Psychiatry*, 1974, *31*, 829–838.

Dahlberg, C. C. Sexual behavior in the drug culture. *Medical Aspects of Human Sexuality*, 1971, *5*, 64–71.

Gay, G. R., Newmeyer, J. A., Perry, M., Johnson, G., and Kurland, M. Love and Haight: The sensuous hippie revisited. Drug/sex practices in San Francisco, 1980–81. *Journal of Psychoactive Drugs*, 1982, *14*, 111–123.

Gay, G. R., Newmeyer, J. A., Elion, R. A., and Wieder, S. The sensuous hippie: Drug/sex practices in the Haight-Ashbury. *Drug Forum*, 1977, *6*, 27–47.

Gay, G. R. and Sheppard, C. W. Sex-crazed dope fiends—Myth or reality? *Drug Forum*, 1973, *2*, 125–140.

Hampton, W. H. Observed psychiatric reactions following use of amphetamine and amphetamine-like substances. *Bull. N.Y. Academy of Medicine,* 1961, *37,* 172.

Jackson, B. and Reed, A. Another absolute amphetamine. *Journal of the American Medical Association,* 1970, *211,* 830.

Korns, H. M., and Randall, W. L. Benzedrine and paredrine in the treatment of orthostatic hypotension, with supplementary case report. *Annals of Internal Medicine,* 1938, *12,* 253–255.

Leavitt, F. I. Drug-induced modifications in sexual behavior and open field locomotion of male rats. *Physiology and Behavior,* 1969, *4,* 677, 683.

Loewe, S. Ejaculation induced by drug action. *Archives Internationales de Pharmacodynamic et de Therapie,* 1938, *60* (1), 37–46.

Monroe, R. R. and Drell, H. J. Oral use of stimulants obtained from inhalers. *Journal of the American Medical Association,* 1947, *135,* 909.

Nail, R. L., Gunderson, E., and Kolb, D. Motives for drug use among light and heavy users. *The Journal of Nervous and Mental Disease,* 1974, *2,* 131–136.

Norman, H. J., and Shea, H. T. Acute hallucinosis as a complication of addiction to amphetamine sulfate. *New England Journal of Medicine,* 1945, *233,* 270.

Parr, D. Sexual aspects of drug abuse in narcotic addicts. *British Journal of Addiction,* 1976, *71,* 261–268.

Schick, J. F. E., Smith, D. E., and Wesson, D. R. An analysis of amphetamine toxicity and patterns of use. *Journal of Psychedelic Drugs,* 1972, *5,* 113, 124, 125, 128, 129.

Schilder, P. Psychological effects of benzedrine sulfate. *Journal Nervous and Mental Disease,* 1938, *87,* 584.

Schiorring, E. Changes in individual and social behavior induced by amphetamine and related compounds in monkeys and man. In *Cocaine and Other Stimulants,* E. H. Ellinwood and M. M. Kibley (Eds.), Plenum Press, N.Y., 1977, 481–522.

Scott, P. D. and Willcox, D. R. C. Delinquency and the amphetamines. *British Journal of Psychiatry,* 1965, *111,* 865–875.

Smith, D. E., Buxton, M. E., and Dammann, G. Amphetamine Abuse and Sexual Dysfunction: Clinical and Research Considerations. In *Amphetamine use, misuse, and abuse: proceedings of the national amphetamine conference,* Ed. D. E. Smith, D. R. Wesson, M. E. Buxton, R. B. Seymour, J. T. Ungerleider, J. P. Morgan, A. J. Mandell, G. Jara (Eds.), Boston, Massachusetts, G. K. Hall & Company, 1978, 228–48.

Soulairac, M. L. Etude experimentale des regulations hormono-nerveuses du comportement sexuel du rat male. *Ann. Endoc.* (Paris), 1963, *24,* 1–98.

Stoffer, S. S., Sapira, J. D., Tweeddale, D. W., and Meketon, B. F. Evaluation of D-amphetamine in menstruation. *American Journal of Obstetrics and Gynecology,* 1969, *105,* 989–990.

Waud, S. P. The effects of toxic doses of benzyl methyl carbinamine (Benzedrine) in man. *Journal of the American Medical Association,* 1938, *110,* 206.

Weil, A. T. Letters from Andrew Weil. *Journal of Psychedelic Drugs,* 1976, *4,* 335–337.

Chapter 3

Amyl Nitrite

The volatile nitrites, such as amyl nitrite, are liquids which are inhaled and have been used in medical practice since the mid-1800s in the treatment of angina pectoris. Prior to 1968, these substances were available without prescription. After 1968, these substances were also used as room odorizers and as such could be obtained without prescription. These products are marketed under several different trade names which indicate the intent for which they are actually sold, e.g., Heart On, Aroma of Men, Rush. These products come in fragile 10-30 ml bottles ("poppers") which are easily "popped" or "snapped" so that the contents can be inhaled.

The basis for their medical use is the vasodilation they produce which results in decreased blood pressure. The subjective effects of these substances include increased awareness, alterations in mood, and dizziness.

In the last several years, volatile nitrites have also begun to be used for sexual enhancement, especially among homosexuals. In 1979, Lowry (1979) reported that annual sales of volatile nitrites were over 250,000,000 doses and contended that amyl and isobutyl nitrite have "become (the) leading recreational drugs in this country." In their initial report of patients at the Haight-Ashbury Free Clinic who were questioned with respect to their drug-sex practices, all stated having used these drugs during intercourse. In a subsequent study, Gay and co-workers (1982) noted that over one-third of both heterosexual and homosexual respondents claimed using nitrites for sexual purposes. In a manual on homosexual sex, *The Joy of Gay Sex*, Silverstein (1977) comments that amyl nitrite "has passed into every corner of gay life."

ANECDOTAL REPORTS

Anecdotal reports support the use of volatile nitrites for sexual enhancement. Gay and co-workers (1973, 1982) quote users as saying:

> "I felt like a car with brand new super-chargers and barrels added" (1973, p. 115).
>
> "Poppers are a lust drug" (1982, p. 115).
>
> "Amyl gives an engorgement of my genitals; a sense of merging with my partner, it heightens my body response and body rhythm. It plays a primary role in the erotic turn-on while I'm able to space-off into the complete pleasure of sensuality" (1982, p. 115).

Lowry (1979a) quotes one user as follows:

> "It's like being shot through the stars in a rocket. The orgasm is truly awesome. I can feel my whole body accelerate; my climax keeps building up; all the rest of the world just disappears and it seems to go on forever. Words are no good to tell you how I get lost in my lover and the sensations. My inhibitions evaporate and almost every kind of sex seems possible and desirable. My whole body streams and throbs . ." (p. 19).

SURVEY STUDIES

Few studies have been reported concerning use of volatile nitrites for sexual enhancement despite the apparent popularity of these drugs.

Lowry (1979a,b) sent questionnaires to known nitrite users in California and received 255 replies, most of which were from men.

Average use was 2.3 times per week. Ninety-three percent of the respondents claimed to have experienced orgasm while under the influence of these drugs. About 20% claimed the drugs facilitated sexual activities previously experienced as negative, such as anal intercourse. About 10% of the respondents reported temporary loss of erection.

In their study of patients at the Haight-Ashbury Free Medical Clinic and Heroin Detoxification Clinic, Gay *et al.* (1977) found that amyl nitrite was not frequently used "to make sex better"—marihuana, tobacco, cocaine, alcohol, amphetamines, barbiturates being preferred much more. Amyl nitrite was also rated fairly low as enhancing sexual experience, but the authors suggest that this may have been due to the relative inexperience of their subjects (mainly heterosexuals) with the drug.

In a subsequent study (Gay *et al.*, 1982) in which a nonpatient population including both heterosexuals and homosexuals was interviewed, volatile nitrites were cited as the third most preferred drug (after marihuana and cocaine) used "to make sex better." More homosexuals and bisexuals used nitrites to make sex better (87% and 75%, respectively), compared to heterosexuals (12%).

When asked to compare nitrites versus cocaine for their ability to increase sexual pleasure, homosexuals and bisexuals rated nitrites above cocaine. In noting these differences, Gay *et al.* (1982) posed the interesting question of why heterosexuals who had used nitrites rated them so much lower than homosexuals.

Goode and Troiden (1979) interviewed 150 homosexual men with respect to their sexual activities and drug use. A list of drugs, including amyl nitrite, was included in a questionnaire and respondents were asked to note which ones they had taken for nonmedical purposes, and how often. Respondents were then divided into groups on the basis of regularity of use of amyl nitrite.

Compared to non-users, regular users (once a week or more) were considerably more likely to have had sex with a greater number of partners (17% vs. 38%); to have engaged in group sex more often (65% vs. 96%); to have engaged in sex with the same partner less often (22% vs. 44%); and were more likely to have

engaged in sex at least three times a week during the preceding
years (33% vs. 67%).

SUMMARY AND CONCLUSIONS

The popularity of volatile nitrites as enticers of sex has increased markedly in recent years, but the popularity is mainly
confined to homosexuals and bisexuals. At present, there is only
speculation as to any pharmacological basis for this preference.
Goode and Troiden (1979) contend that the individual who is at-
tracted to the use of amyl nitrite is also more likely to be one who is
more likely to engage in unconventional sex practices to begin
with, and use of the drug and deviant sex practices are both influ-
enced by area of residence.

The pharmacological basis for nitrite use may be due to
smooth muscle relaxation and resulting vasodilation in genitourinary vessels which these substances also produce (Louria, 1970), or
a relaxation of the anal sphincter, facilitating anal intercourse
among homosexuals (Labataille, 1975), or psychologically, an altered perception of sensory experience (Lowry, 1979).

With respect to the latter possibility, Lowry notes that "a whiff
of amyl nitrite, as used in clinical and diagnostic settings, is perceived as mildly unpleasant with feelings of dizziness, nausea,
flushed skin, and pounding heart; but in a setting of affection and
passion, taken about 30 seconds before orgasm, there can be a
strong enhancement of perceptions (Loury, 1979a, p. 19). This interpretation emphasizes the important factors of "set" and
"setting."

Although used as a sexual stimulant, amyl nitrite has also
been used clinically to reduce penile tumescence (Welti and
Brodsky, 1980). In this report, penile erection occurred after anesthesia. One inhalent capsule of amyl nitrite was then placed into
the breathing bag and within four minutes, penile detumescence
and eventual flaccidity developed. The authors suggested that this
effect may have been due to a decrease in blood pressure which

"may mimic the sympathetic discharge that occurs during orgasm, which precipitates arteriolas constriction and termination of erection."

References

Gay, G. R., Newmeyer, J. A., Perry, M., Johnson, G., and Kurland, M. Love and Haight: The sensuous hippie revisited. Drug/sex practices in San Francisco, 1980–81. *Journal of Psychoactive Drugs*, 1982, *14*, 111–123.

Gay, G. R., Newmeyer, J. A., Elion, R. A., and Weider, S. The sensuous hippie: Drug/sex practices in the Haight-Ashbury. *Drug Forum*, 1977, *6*, 27–47.

Gay, G. R. and Sheppard, C. W. Sex-crazed dope fiends—Myth or reality? *Drug Forum*, 1973, *2*, 125–140.

Goode, E. and Troiden, R. R. Amyl nitrite use among homosexual men. *American Psychiatric Association*, 1979, *136*, 1067–69.

Labataille, L. Amyl nitrite employed in homosexual relations. *Medical Aspects of Human Sexuality*, 1975, *9*, 122.

Louria, D. B. Sexual use of amyl nitrite. *Medical Aspects of Human Sexuality*, 1970, *4*, 89.

Lowry, T. P. Amyl nitrates: An old high comes back to visit. *Behavioral Medicine*, 1979a, *6*, 19–21.

Lowry, T. P. The volatile nitrites as sexual drugs: A user survey. *Journal of Sex Education and Therapy*, 1979b, *1*, 8.

Silverstein, C. and White, E. *The joy of gay sex*. New York, Crown Publishers, 1977.

Welti, R. S. and Brodsky, J. B. Treatment of intraoperative penile tumescence. *Journal of Urology*, 1980, *124*, 925–926.

Chapter 4

Antidepressants

Antidepressant drugs are usually divided into two main categories, the tricyclic antidepressants and the monoamine oxidase inhibitors (MAOIs). The former are by far the most widely administered of the two.

The tricyclic antidepressants are so called because of their basic three-ring structure. Although they are also similar in structure to antipsychotic compounds such as chlorpromazine, they do not possess antipsychotic activity. It was actually as a result of trying to synthesize a variant of chlorpromazine that imipramine, the prototypic tricyclic antidepressant, was produced. Although imipramine was not found to be useful in treating schizophrenics, it was found effective in treating depression.

The mechanism of action of the tricyclics involves blocking reuptake of norepinephrine (but not dopamine) and serotonin into presynaptic terminals. As a result, these neurotransmitters act at receptor sites for a longer time than would otherwise be the case.

The other class of antidepressants, the MOAIs, accomplish the same effect by inhibiting the actions of monoamine oxidase, the enzyme which breaks down norepinephrine and serotonin.

Although antidepressants act through mechanisms similar to those that underlie the actions of the amphetamines, antidepressants do not affect mood unless they are used consistently for several weeks. Because effects are not immediate, these drugs are not abused.

In evaluating the effects of these drugs on sexuality, the fact that decreased sexual arousal is a frequent characteristic of depression should be kept in mind. Drugs which cause increased sexual arousal in people with depression should therefore be evaluated in the context of this disorder. For instance, any increase in sexual arousal may have resulted from a general improvement in mood rather than any specific effect of the drug. Likewise, any reported decrease in sexual arousal or function may already have occurred prior to drug treatment but may inadvertently be attributed to such treatment.

MALE SEXUALITY

Beaumont (1973) reported that the tricyclic clomipramine increased sexual arousal in 10 of 19 depressed males and 21 of 35 depressed women. However, reports of decreased sexual arousal in conjunction with use of tricyclic antidepressants, such as imipramine (Couper-Smartt & Rodham, 1973), amitriptyline (Hekimian *et al.*, 1978), and amoxapine (Schwarcz, 1982), tend to be more common. Monoamine oxidase inhibitors (MAOIs) such as tranylcypramine have been reported to cause increased sexual arousal at a dose of 20 mg/kg a day (Simpson *et al.*, 1965). Another MAOI, phenelzine, however, produced decreased sexual arousal (Friedman *et al.*, 1978).

Sexual dysfunction occurs much more commonly in connection with the tricyclics than does inhibition of sexual arousal. Erectile dysfunction occurred in 2 out of 3 patients treated with imipramine by Everett (1975) and has also been noted in conjunction with amitriptyline medication (Couper-Smartt & Rodham, 1973). Simpson and co-workers (1975) reported that tranylcypromine produced impotence at a dose of 20 mg/kg but that this effect was not observed when the dose was lowered to 10 mg/kg. Kulik and

Wilbur (1982) report a case in which a patient receiving amoxapine experienced no loss of libido or erectile function but when ejaculation occurred, it "dribbled" out. This ejaculatory dysfunction disappeared 3 to 4 days after drug treatment was discontinued.

Inhibition of ejaculation has also been frequently reported in patients receiving imipramine (Couper-Smartt & Rodham, 1973; Simpson *et al.*, 1965) and other tricyclic antidepressants (Beaumont, 1973; Couper-Smartt & Rodham, 1973; Kulik and Wilbur, 1982; Nininger, 1978; Simpson *et al.*, 1965). There are also reports of painful ejaculation associated with use of these drugs (Simpson *et al.*, 1976). As a result of their effects on ejaculation, tricyclic antidepressants have been used clinically to delay premature ejaculation (Eaton, 1973).

EFFECTS ON SPERM

Blair and his co-workers (1962) reported that phenelzine increased sperm count and sperm motility in men. In two of the three men tested, sperm counts increased by over 100 percent. Likewise, Davis and co-workers (1966) observed a significant increase in sperm count in a group of men with low sperm counts. In contrast to MOAIs, tricyclic antidepressants do not affect sperm count or motility *in vivo* (Levin *et al.*, 1981; Simpson *et al.*, 1965) but do inhibit sperm motility *in vitro* (Levin *et al.*, 1981).

FEMALE SEXUALITY

There have been a few reports of the effects of antidepressants on sexual arousal or function in women. Two out of four of the female patients treated by Wyatt and his co-workers (1971) with phenelzine (60 mg/kg a day), a MAIO inhibitor, reported difficulty in achieving orgasm. Three additional such cases were noted by Lesko and her co-workers (1982). Moss (1983), Pohl (1983), and Barton (1979) each noted anorgasmia in one of their patients receiving phenelzine. Tricyclic antidepressants such as imipramine and clomipramine have also been associated with anorgasmia in women (Beaumont, 1973; Sovner, 1983) as has amoxapine (Shen, 1982).

Studies in Animals

Leavitt (1969) administered tranylcypromine (2.0 and 4.0 mg/kg) to sexually experienced male rats placed with estrus females. Drug treatment did not significantly affect sexual behavior in these males.

Summary and Conclusions

There is considerable evidence that antidepressants can decrease sexual arousal and function. However, in many cases these problems may be due more to the underlying depression than to the drugs used to treat this condition. Since tricyclic antidepressants affect adrenergic and cholinergic mechanisms, effects on sexual arousal and function could be the result of actions at many different sites, and while several explanations have been suggested (Kulik & Wilbur, 1982) none of these can account for the reported effects without reservation.

References

Barton, J. L. Orgasmic inhibition by phenelzine. *American Journal of Psychiatry*, 1979, *136*, 1616–1617.

Beaumont, G. Sexual side effects of clomipramine (Anafranil). *Journal of Internal Medicine and Research*, 1973, *1*, 469–473.

Blair, J. H., Simpson, G. M., and Kline, N. S. Monoamine oxidase inhibitors and sperm production. *Journal of the American Medical Association*, 1962, *181*, 192–193.

Couper-Smartt, J. D. and Rodham, R. A technique for surveying side effects of tricyclic drugs with reference to reported sexual effects. *Journal of Internal Medicine and Research*, 1973, *1*, 473–476.

Davis, J., Clyman, M. J., Decker, A., Bronstein, S., and Roland, M. Effect of phenelzine on semen in infertility: A preliminary report. *Fertility and Sterility*, 1966, *17*, 221–225.

Eaton, H. Clomipramine (Anafranil) in the treatment of premature ejaculation. *Journal of Internal Medicine and Research*, 1973, *1*, 432–434.

Everett, H. C. The use of bethanechol chloride with tricyclic antidepressants. *American Journal of Psychiatry*, 1975, *132*, 1202–1204.

Friedman, S., Kantor, I., and Sobel, S. A follow-up study on the chemotherapy of neurodermatitis with monoamine oxidase. *Journal of Nervous and Mental Diseases*, 1978, *166*, 349–357.

Hekimian, L. J., Friedhoff, A. J., and Deever, E. A comparison of the onset of action and therapeutic efficacy of amoxapine and amitriptyline. *Journal of Clinical Psychiatry*, 1978, *39*, 633–637.

Kulik, F. A. and Wilbur, R. Case report of painful ejaculation as a side effect of amoxapine. *American Journal of Psychiatry*, 1982, *139*, 234–235.

Leavitt, F. I. Drug-induced modifications in sexual behavior and open field locomotion of male rats. *Physiology and Behavior*, 1969, *4*, 677–683.

Lesko, L. M., Stotland, N. L., and Segraves, R. T. Three cases of female anorgasmia associated with MAOIs. *American Journal of Psychiatry*, 1982, *139*, 1353–1354.

Levin, R. M., Amsterdam, J. D., Winokur, A., and Wein, A. J. Effects of psychotropic drugs on human sperm motility. *Fertility and Sterility*, 1981, *36*, 503–506.

Moss, H. B. More cases of anorgasmia after MOAI treatment. *American Journal of Psychiatry*, 1983, *140*, 266–267.

Nininger, J. E. Inhibition of ejaculation by amitriptyline. *American Journal of Psychiatry*, 1978, *135*, 750–751.

Pohl, R. Anorgasmia caused by MAOIs. *American Journal of Psychiatry*, 1983, *140*, 510.

Schwarcz, G. Case report of inhibition of ejaculation and retrograde ejaculation as side effects of amoxapine. *American Journal of Psychiatry*, 1982, *139*, 233–234.

Shen, W. W. Female orgasmic inhibition by amoxapine. *American Journal of Psychiatry*, 1982, *139*, 1220.

Simpson, G. M., Blair, J. H., and Amuso, D. Effects of antidepressants on genitourinary function. *Diseases of the Nervous System*, 1965, *26*, 787–789.

Sovner, R. Anorgasmia associated with imipramine but not desipramine: Case report. *Journal of Clinical Psychiatry*, 1983, *44*, 345–346.

Wyatt, R. J., Fram, D. H., and Buchbinder, R. Treatment of intractable narcolepsy with a monoamine oxidase inhibitor. *New England Journal of Medicine*, 1971, *285*, 987–988.

Chapter 5

Antipsychotics

Antipsychotic drugs or major tranquilizers as they are also called, are primarily used for psychotic disorders such as schizophrenia and have virtually no potential for abuse or recreational usage.

This class of drugs is divided into three different categories depending on their structure. One of these are the derivatives of phenothiazine, the prototype of which is chlorpromazine (Thorazine). Chlorpromazine was initially regarded as an antihistamine but clinical testing revealed it to have potent tranquilizing properties in management of previously unmanageable psychotics. Associated with this tranquilizing action, phenothiazines decrease general motor activity. At high doses they can induce cataleptic-like effects. Associated with this effect on activity are characteristic extrapyramidal side effects such as muscle spasms and speech difficulties.

A major site of action for these drugs in the brain is the reticular activating system, and particularly the ascending system which receives sensory input. Phenothiazines have been found to exert a blockade of alpha-adrenergic receptors in the autonomic nervous system and may possibly affect adrenergic pathways in the reticular activating system in the same way.

A second category of antipsychotics are the butyrophenones,

79

the prototype of which is haloperidol (Haldol). The mechanism of action of these drugs appears to involve blockade of dopamine receptors.

The third class of antipsychotics are the rauwolfia alkaloids of which reserpine is the prototype. These drugs produce long-lasting depletion of norepinephrine from neurons and they impair binding of newly synthesized amines. The result is tantamount to a blockade of adrenergic receptors.

Since antipsychotics exert wide-ranging effects on neuronal transmission in the central and peripheral nervous systems, it is not surprising that use of these drugs is accompanied by sexual dysfunction. Such dysfunction has primarily been documented in men and therefore much of the following survey will address these side effects primarily with respect to male sexuality.

MALE SEXUALITY

Decreased sexual arousal is a common side-effect of antipsychotic drugs (e.g., Freyhan, 1961; Greenberg, 1971; Haider, 1966; Kotin *et al.*, 1976). Greenberg (1971) found that this effect was dose-related. Doses of 1200 mg/kg of chlorpromazine decreased sexual arousal considerably. At a dose of 400 mg/kg, sexual arousal was restored, although other aspects of sexual function were still impaired.

A very common side effect of these drugs is erectile impotence. About 40–60% of all patients receiving thioridiazine (Mellaril) report this effect (e.g., Blair & Simpson, 1966; Haider, 1966; Kotin *et al.*, 1976). Other antipsychotics also produce erectile dysfunction but the incidence is not as high. In one comparative study, Kotin *et al.* (1976) reported a 44% incidence of erectile impotence in patients receiving Mellaril compared to a 19% incidence for patients receiving other forms of antipsychotics. In addition, 35% of the patients receiving Mellaril reported difficulty in maintaining erection compared to 1% for those receiving other antipsychotics.

Greenberg (1971) reported a dose-response relation between chlorpromazine and erectile impotence. At doses of 1000 mg/kg erectile dysfunction occurred but when the dosage was reduced to 600 mg/kg erectile dysfunction was ameliorated.

In contrast to these reports of erectile impotence, however, there are also reports of priapism associated with antipsychotic medication (e.g., Appell *et al.*, 1977; Gottlieb & Lustberg, 1977). This discrepancy in action has not been explained.

The most commonly reported sexual dysfunction associated with antipsychotics is ejaculatory dysfunction. This has been noted especially in conjunction with thioridazine (e.g., Blair & Simpson, 1966; Clein, 1962; Haider, 1966; Kotin *et al.*, 1976; Shader, 1967), but has also been reported in connection with other antipsychotics (e.g., Blair & Simpson, 1966; Greenberg, 1971).

EFFECTS ON HORMONES

Studies examining the effects of antipsychotics on testosterone levels have been inconsistent in their results. For example, there are reports that antipsychotics increase testosterone levels (Brambilla *et al.*, 1975), do not affect testosterone levels (Arato *et al.*, 1979; Cotes *et al.*, 1978), or decrease testosterone levels (Beaumont *et al.*, 1974) during drug maintenance. Brambilla *et al.* (1975) administered haloperidol for 30 days to schizophrenics. Testosterone levels did not change during drug treatment.

Similarly, reports of changes in levels of plasma LH also range from increases (Brambilla *et al.*, 1975) to decreases (Brown, 1981) to no change (Rubin *et al.*, 1976). Some antipsychotics such as thioridazine may also have a greater effect on testosterone and LH levels than other hormones (Brown, 1981).

In contrast to these inconsistencies, there is a consensus that antipsychotics cause serum prolactin levels to be increased (Collu *et al.*, 1975; Gruen *et al.*, 1978; Martin du Pan *et al.*, 1976; Meltzer & Fang, 1976; Siris *et al.*, 1980).

Effects on Sperm

Chlorpromazine, at low concentrations, has been found to reduce sperm motility *in vitro* (Levin *et al.*, 1981). Whether a comparable effect occurs *in vivo* is unknown.

Effects in Animals

Zimbardo and Barry (1958) injected male rats with chlorpromazine (1 mg/kg) and placed them with females in estrus. The drug did not affect the number of males that copulated or ejaculated, but it did increase latencies to mount and ejaculate. Gillett (1960) tested male rats with a higher dose of chlorpromazine (2.5 mg/kg) and observed a decrease in the number of copulations prior to ejaculation, but no effect on copulatory attempts.

Cranston (1958) added chlorpromazine to the diet given to female mice to determine if the drug would affect estrus cycles. A decrease in the number of estrus cycles ranging from 46% to 70% occurred depending on the amount of chlorpromazine in the diet.

Summary and Conclusions

Erectile and ejaculatory failure are commonly associated with antipsychotic medication. However, many patients receiving such drugs may have pre-existing conditions which account for their sexual dysfunction. For example, schizophrenia is associated with decreased basal levels of testosterone (Brambilla *et al.*, 1975) and LH (Jonstone *et al.*, 1977). Failure to compare predrug and postdrug levels of hormones may thus result in inaccurate assessments of drug effects.

On the other hand, antipsychotics interfere with dopamine transmission (Van Pragg, 1977) and since dopamine appears to be involved in sexual function (see Introduction), dysfunction may be mediated through dopaminergic mechanisms. One such mechanism may involve dopaminergic mediation of prolactin levels. The increase in prolactin levels produced by these drugs is believed to occur as a result of blockade of dopamine receptors. Hyperprolactinemia has been associated with decreased sexual arousal and erectile dysfunction (Martin du Pan *et al.*, 1976).

Shader (1967) has suggested that antipsychotics inhibited ejaculation as a result of their alpha-adrenergic receptor blocking action. This same mechanism has also been suggested to account for the priapism induced by antipsychotics (Dorman & Schmidt, 1976).

References

Appell, R. A., Shield, D. E., and McGuire, E. J. Thioridazine-induced priapism. *British Journal of Urology*, 1977, *49*, 160–164.

Arato, M., Erdo, S. A., and Polgar, M. Endocrinological changes in patients with sexual dysfunction under long-term neuroleptic treatment. *Neuropsychopharmakologie*, 1979, *12*, 426–432.

Beaumont, P. J. V., Corker, C. S., Friesen, H. G., Kolakowska, F. T., Mandelbrote, B. M., Marshall, S., Murrey, M. A. F., and Wiles, D. M. The effects of phenothiazines on endocrine function: II. Effects in men and post-menopausal women. *British Journal of Psychiatry*, 1974, *124*, 420–430.

Blair, J. H. and Simpson, G. M. Effect of antipsychotic drugs on reproductive dysfunctions. *Diseases of the Nervous System*, 1966, *27*, 645–647.

Brambilla, F., Guerrini, A., Guastall, A., Rovere, C., and Riggle, F. Neuroendocrine effects of haloperidol therapy in chronic schizophrenia. *Psychopharmacologia*, 1975, *44*, 17–22.

Clein, L. Thioridazine and ejaculation. *British Medical Journal*, 1962, *2*, 548–549.

Collu, R., Jequier, J. C., and Laboeuf, G. Endocrine effects of pimozide, a specific dopaminergic blocker. *Journal of Clinical Endocrinology and Metabolism*, 1975, *41*, 981–984.

Cotes, P. M., Crow, T. J., Johnstone, E. C., Bartlett, W., and Bourne, R. C. Neuroendocrine changes in acute schizophrenia as a function of clinical state and neuroleptic medication. *Psychological Medicine*, 1978, *8*, 657–665.

Cranston, E. M. Effect of tranquilizers and other agents on sexual cycle of mice. *Proceedings of the Society of Experimental Biology and Medicine*, 1958, *98*, 320–322.

Dorman, B. W. and Schmidt, J. D. Association of priapism in phenothiazine therapy. *Journal of Urology*, 1976, *116*, 51–53.

Freyhan, F. A. Loss of ejaculation during Mellaril treatment. *American Journal of Psychiatry*, 1961, *118*, 171–172.

Gillett, E. Effects of chlorpromazine and d-lysergic acid diethylamide on sex behavior of male rats. *Proceedings of the Society of Experimental Biology and Medicine*, 1960, *103*, 392–394.

Gottlieb, J. I. and Lustberg, T. Phenothiazine-induced priapism: A case report. *American Journal of Psychiatry*, 1977, *134*, 1445–1446.

Greenberg, H. Inhibition of ejaculation by chlorpromazine. *Journal of Nervous and Mental Diseases*, 1971, *152*, 364–366.

Gruen, P. H., Sachar, E. J., and Altman, N. Relations of plasma prolactin to clinical response in schizophrenic patients. *Archives of General Psychiatry*, 1978, *35*, 1222–1227.

Haider, I. Thioridazine and sexual dysfunctions. *International Journal of Neuropsychiatry*, 1966, *5*, 255–257.

Jonstone, E. C., Crow, T. J., and Mashiter, K. Anterior pituitary hormone secretion in chronic schizophrenia—a approach to neurohumoral mechanisms. *Psychological Medicine*, 1977, *7*, 223–228.

Kotin, J., Wibert, D. E., Verbug, D., and Soldinger, S. M. Thioridazine and sexual dysfunction. *American Journal of Psychiatry*, 1976, *133*, 82–85.

Levin, R. M., Amsterdam, J. D., Winokur, A., and Wein, A. J. Effects of psychotropic drugs on human sperm motility. *Fertility and Sterility*, 1981, *36*, 503–506.

Mann, T. Effects of pharmacological agents on male sexual functions. *Journal of Reproduction and Fertility*, 1968, *Supplement 4*, 101–114.

Martin du Pan, R., Baumann, P., Magrini, G., and Felber, J. P. Neuroendocrine effects of chronic neuroleptic therapy in male psychiatric patients. *Psychoneuroendocrinology*, 1976, *3*, 245–252.

Meltzer, H. Y. and Fang, V. S. The effect of neuroleptics on serum prolactin in schizophrenic patients. *Archives of General Psychiatry*, 1976, *33*, 279–286.

Rubin, R. T., Poland, R. E., O'Connor, D., Gouin, P. R., and Tower, B. B. Selective neuroendocrine effects of low-dose haloperidol in normal adult men. *Psychopharmacology*, 1976, *47*, 135–140.

Schader, R. I. Sexual dysfunction associated with thioridazine hydrochloride. *Journal of the American Medical Association*, 1967, *28*, 240–244.

Siris, S. G., Siris, E. S., Van Kammen, D. P., Docherty, J. P., Alexander, P. E., and Bunney, W. E. Effects of dopamine blockade on gonadotropins and testosterone in men. *American Journal of Psychiatry*, 1980, *137*, 211–214.

Van Praag, H. M. The significance of dopamine for the mode of action of neuroleptics and the pathogenesis of schizophrenia. *British Journal of Psychiatry*, 1977, *130*, 463–474.

Zimbardo, P. G. and Barry, H. Effects of caffeine and chlorpromazine on the sexual behavior of male rats. *Science*, 1958, *127*, 84–85.

Chapter 6

Barbiturates

Barbiturates are sedative and hypnotic drugs. At low doses (about 50 mg), they produce a sedating or calming effect on anxiety, mild euphoria, relaxation, impairment of memory, and a sense of release from inhibitions. At moderative doses (about 150 mg), they produce an intensification of many of the effects obtained at lower doses and in some people a paradoxical excitement and hostility rather than relaxation. At higher doses they produce drowsiness. Tolerance develops very rapidly to these drugs and tolerance to barbiturates results in cross tolerance to alcohol. Physical dependence on barbiturates also occurs and abstinence can precipitate dangerous withdrawal reactions.

Although the brain is the primary site of action, these drugs also affect other organs, especially the liver and heart. In the brain, the primary sites of action are the systems that control arousal— the reticular activating system and the diffuse thalamic projection system. The effects of these drugs are not dependent on any single specific action at the cellular level. Among the proposed mechanisms are interference with cellular oxidation and depression of pre- and post-synaptic neurotransmitter function, especially that involving GABA.

MALE SEXUALITY

On the basis of their first study of 50 patients at the Haight Ashbury Free Clinic, Gay and Sheppard (1973) commented that "in the hierarchy of the drug-using subculture, true barb freaks are not highly regarded, either as lovers or otherwise" (p. 131). The authors also comment that while barbiturates were sometimes taken by couples to "relax," libido and performance generally decrease. When asked to rate the effects of barbiturates on enhancement of sexual pleasure, respondents rated barbiturates as having no augmenting effect.

In their study of drug users in the navy, Nail and co-workers (1974) reported that increased sexuality was not among the reasons cited for barbiturate use.

Barbiturates were also rated very poorly in terms of drugs used "to make sex better" in a second study reported by Gay and his co-workers (1977). Overall, barbiturates were rated second last and just slightly above heroin in terms of effects on sexuality, and in terms of enhancing libido or sexual performance. Barbiturates were never chosen in preference to engaging in sex or for use during intercourse. Negative attributes associated with usage include loss of erection, difficulty maintaining erection, and difficulty in achieving ejaculation.

Similar findings were noted in Gay *et al.*'s (1982) study of nonpatient "gourmet" drug users. In response to a question of which drugs respondents chose "to make sex better," less than 10% of the 102 respondents cited barbiturates. Barbiturates were also cited second last among drugs rated for increasing sexual pleasure.

STUDIES IN ANIMALS

Crowley and co-workers (1974) intravenously administered sodium pentobarbital (0 to 1 mg/kg) to adult male monkeys living in a colony of about 30 adults. Although other drugs, e.g., amphetamine, ethanol, affected sexual behavior in these animals, pentobarbital had no significant effects in this regard.

Van der Schoot (1980) reported that pentobarbital inhibited sexually receptive behavior (lordosis) in female rats with 5-day estrus cycles on the day after injection. In contrast, all females with 4-day cycles exhibited receptive behavior the day after the second injection of pentobarbital.

EFFECTS ON SPERM

Only one study was located in which barbiturate effects on sperm were noted. In this study by Levin and co-workers (1981), barbital did not affect *in vitro* motility of human sperm.

EFFECTS ON HORMONES

Testosterone

Linnoila and co-workers (1980) compared the effects of pentobarbital (100 mg capsules) to placebo for its effects on serum plasma testosterone levels in men. Treatments were administered "double blind" so that neither the experimenters nor subjects knew the drug condition. Pentobarbital did not significantly affect plasma testosterone levels.

Zaidi and co-workers (1982) reported that pentobarbital anesthesia (12 mg/kg/hr) increased serum testosterone levels 4-fold in male monkeys. The measured testosterone levels were associated with a 13-fold increase on production rate of testosterone, and a 2-fold increase in metabolic clearance.

Franz and Longcope (1979) likewise noted increased serum testosterone levels following barbiturate-induced anesthesia in monkeys, although the magnitude of the increase was considerably lower than that observed by Zaidi *et al.* (1982).

In contrast to these observations in monkeys, Carstinsen and co-workers (1974) noted a significant decrease in plasma testosterone levels and testosterone production rates lasting as long as 24 hours after barbiturate-induced anesthesia in dogs.

In rats, Cicero and Badger (1977) reported pentobarbital (40 mg/kg) did not affect testosterone levels up to one hour after injection. Between two and four hours after injection, however, testosterone levels fell by about 40% compared to controls and returned to control levels by six hours after injection.

Luteinizing Hormone

Zaidi and co-workers (1982) reported that pentobarbital-induced anesthesia caused a significant increase in serum LH levels in male monkeys that preceded a subsequent increase in testosterone levels in the same animals.

Considerably more attention has been devoted to barbiturate effects on LH in female animals. An early review of this literature can be found in Cicero and Badger (1977).

Barbiturates reliably inhibit the spontaneous rise in plasma LH and inhibit its release during proestrus in the rat (e.g., Beattie *et al.*, 1973; Blake, 1974a; Van der Schoot, 1980). This effect does not occur at doses of pentobarbital of 25 mg/kg or less but delays in release of about 3 hours compared to spontaneous release may still occur. Similar effects have been observed after administration of pentobarbital. When phenobarbital was administered in conjunction with LH-releasing hormone (100 μg), pituitary release of LH was actually increased (Blake, 1974a; Wedig and Gay, 1973).

Likewise, Blake (1974b) reported that neither phenobarbital nor pentobarbital was able to suppress LH-RH-induced release of LH ovariectomized rats. The observations indicate that barbiturates do not inhibit LH release in the pituitary. Blake (1974b) also found that barbiturates inhibited LH release even after partial or total deafferentation of the medical basal hypothalamus–median eminence (MBH) indicating that the site of action of barbiturates on LH release is in the hypothalamus.

Rance and Barraclaugh (1981) reported that phenobarbital did not prevent the use in LH–RH levels in the median eminence. Barbiturates also do not affect release of LH–RH from the median eminence, but portal plasma LH–RH levels do not increase concomitantly (Eskay *et al.*, 1977). These results suggest that the suppressant effects of barbiturates in LH are also not due to ME–LHRH accumulation or release.

Hogino (1979) also reported that intramuscular administration of pentobarbital, which produced sedation, suppressed the proestus increase in LH in monkeys.

EFFECTS ON OVULATION

Barbiturates have long been known to be capable of blocking ovulation in animals (e.g., Everett *et al.*, 1949; Everett, 1961, p. 467). Cranston (1958) placed phenobarbital in the diet given to mice. At a concentration of 0.2%, ovulation was completely inhibited. At a concentration of 0.1%, ovulation was inhibited about 40% of the time. Body weight of animals in this study was decreased by less than 1 gram, indicating that the effect was not likely to be due to undernutrition.

This inhibitory effect depends on the length of the reproductive cycle in the rat. In rats with a 4-day cycle, pentobarbital injected at proestrus can delay ovulation by 1 or 2 days (e.g., Butcher *et al.*, 1974; Everett & Sawyer, 1950; Everett *et al.*, 1949; Van der Schoot, 1980). In rats with 5-day cycles, pentobarbital is able to inhibit ovulation completely (Van der Shoot, 1978, 1980).

SUMMARY AND CONCLUSIONS

Little information is available concerning the effects of barbiturates on sexual behavior. In the male, the available data indicate that barbiturates decrease both LH and testosterone levels in animals. Doses of barbiturates that do so, however, are relatively high and no comparable effect has been found in humans at low doses.

In the female, barbiturates can inhibit LH release and can inhibit ovulation. This effect is not due to inhibition of LH release since barbiturates do not inhibit LH release after administration of LH–RH. The site of action appears to be in the hypothalamus since partial or complete deafferentation does not affect the effects of barbiturates on LH.

References

Beattie, C. W., Campbell, C. S., Nequin, L. G., Soyha, L. F., and Schwartz, N. B. Barbiturate blockade of tonic LH secretion in the male and female rat. *Endocrinology*, 1973, *92*, 1630–1638.

Blake, Charles, A. Differentiation between the "Critical Period", the "Activation Period" and the "Potential Activation Period" for neurohumoral stimulation of LH release in proestrous rats. *Endocrinology*, 1974a, *95*, 572.

Blake, Charles A. Localization of the inhibitory actions of ovulation-blocking drugs on release of luteinizing hormone in ovariectomized rats. *Endocrinology*, 1974, *95*, 999.

Butcher, R. L., Collins, W. E., and Fugo, N. W. Altered secretion of gonadotropins and steroids resulting from delayed ovulation in the rat. *Endocrinology*, 1974, *96*, 576–586.

Carstinsen, H., Amer, I., Sodergard, R., and Hietala, S. O. Testosterone binding capacity in relation to the production and metabolism of testosterone in dogs. Experience of a new method. *J. Steroid. Biochem.*, 1974, *5*, 757.

Cicero, T. J. and Badger, T. M. A comparative analysis of the effects of narcotics, alcohol, and the barbiturates on the hypothalamic-pituitary-gonadal axis. *Advances in Experimental Medicine and Biology*, 1977, *85B*, 94–115.

Cranston, E. M. Effect of tranquilizers and other agents on sexual cycle of mice. *Proceedings of the Society for Experimental Biology and Medicine*, 1958, *98*, 320.

Crowley, T. J., Stynes, A. J., Hydinger, M., and Kaufman, I. C. Ethanol, methamphetamine, pentobarbital, morphine, and monkey social behavior. *Archives of General Psychiatry*, 1974, *31*, 829.

Eskay, R. L., Mical, R. S., and Porter, J. C. Relationship between luteinizing hormone releasing hormone concentration in hypophysial portal blood and luteinizing hormone release in intact, castrated, and electrochemically-stimulated rats! *Endocrinology*, 1977, *100*, 263.

Everett, J. W. and Sawyer, C. H. A 24-Hour periodicity in the LH-release apparatus of female rats, disclosed by barbiturate sedation. *Endocrinology*, 1950, *47*, 198–218.

Everett, J. W., Sawyer, C. H., Markee, J. E. A neurogenic timing factor in control of the ovulatory discharge of luteinizing hormone in the cyclic rat. *Endocrinology*, 1949, *44*, 234.

Everett, J. W. In *Sex and internal secretions*, W. C. Young (Ed.), Ed. 3, Vol. 1, Williams and Wilkins, Baltimore, 1961, p. 497.

Franz, C. and Longcope, C. Androgen and estrogen metabolism in male rhesus monkeys. *Endocrinology*, 1979, *105*, 869.

Gay, G. R. and Sheppard, C. W. Sex-crazed dope fiends! Myth or reality. *Drug Forum*, 1973, *2*, 125–140.

Gay, G. R., Newmeyer, J. A., Perry, M., Johnson, G., and Kurland, M. Love and Haight: The sensuous hippie revisited. Drug/sex practices in San Francisco 1980–1981. *Journal of Psychoactive Drugs*, 1982, *14*, 111–123.

Gay, G. R., Newmeyer, J. A., Elion, R. A., and Wieder, S. The sensuous hippie, Part I. *Drug Forum*, 1977, *6*, 27–47.

Hogino, N. Effect of Nembutal on LH release in baboons. *Horm. Metab. Res.*, 1979, *11*, 296.

Levin, R. M., Amsterdam, J. D., Winokur, A., and Wein, A. J. Effects of psychotropic drugs on human sperm motility. *Fertility and Sterility*, 1981, *36*, 503–506.

Linnoila, M., Prinz, P. N., Wonsowicz, C. J., and Leppaluoto, J. Effect of moderate doses of ethanol and phenobarbital on pituitary and thyroid hormones and testosterone. *British Journal of Addiction*, 1980, *75*, 207.

Nail, R. L., Gunderson, E. K. E., and Kolb, D. Motives for drug use among light and heavy users. *Journal of Nervous and Mental Disease*, 1974, *159*, 131–136.

Rance, N. and Barraclough, C. A. Effects of phenobarbital on hypothalamic LHRH and catecholamine turnover rates in proestrous rats. *Proceedings of the Society for Experimental Biology and Medicine*, 1981, *166*, 425.

Van der Schoot, P. Plasma oestradiol and delayed ovulation after administration of sodium pentobarbitone to proestrous 5-day-cycle rats. *Journal of Endocrinology*, 1978, *77*, 325–332.

Van Der Schoot, P. Delay of ovulation in rats with sodium pentobarbitone: Apparent differences between rats with 4- or 5-day reproductive cycles. *Journal of Endocrinology*, 1980, *86*, 451–457.

Wedig, J. H. and Gay, V. L. Potentiation of luteinizing hormone-releasing factor activities following pentobarbital anaesthesia in the steroid-blocked castrated rat. *Proceedings of the Society of Experimental Biological Medicine*, 1973, *144*, 993.

Zaidi, P., Wickings, E. J., and Nieschlag, E. The effects of ketamine HCl and barbiturate anaesthesia on the metabolic clearance and production rates of testosterone in the male rhesus monkey Macaca Mulatta. *Journal of Steroid Biochemistry*, 1982, *16*, 463.

Chapter 7

Benzodiazepines

The benzodiazpines, of which Valium (diazepam) and Librium (chlordiazepoxide) are prototypes, were synthesized in the 1950s and are now the most widely used antianxiety agents currently sold. These drugs reduce anxiety with relatively few side effects in contrast to other tranquillizers. Recent studies have shown there are specific benzodiazepine receptors in the brain and it is likely that the antianxiety effects of these drugs are related to their actions at these receptor sites. In addition to antianxiety properties, these drugs are also muscle relaxants and anticonvulsants.

In general, low doses (5 mg) of these drugs first produce sedation. As the dosage is increased sleep occurs and with even higher doses, stupor. Diazepam in large doses also produces euphoria and is sometimes taken along with alcohol for this purpose. Metabolism occurs via the liver and the half-life of diazepam in the body is about 20–90 hours depending on route of administration. Tolerance develops to chronic use of these drugs and withdrawal symptoms can occur following abstinence.

As a consequence of their antianxiety properties, there is the possibility that these drugs could have a beneficial effect on impaired sexuality if such disorders were psychosomatic in origin, especially where anxiety was an underlying cause.

CLINICAL STUDIES

In one of the earlier clinical reports involving Librium, Usdin (1960) reported that 1 of 32 male patients to whom the drug was given initially complained of drug-induced impotence but this effect disappeared after two weeks of continued treatment. None of the 48 female patients reported any effects on sexuality. Maneksha and Harry (1975) administered lorazepam to a group of patients (N=35) as an adjunct to psychotherapy for sexual disorders. The study was conducted "double-blind" and lorazepam was found to be significantly better than placebo in improving sexual relations. In contrast to these reports, however, Ansari (1976) reported that oxazepam did not affect outcome in men being treated for erectile impotence.

Carney and co-workers (1978) compared the effects of diazepam (10 mg) to testosterone in treatment of sexual responsiveness in women. Both groups also received counselling. The patients were assessed under both conditions in a balanced factorial design. Diazepam did not significantly affect sexuality although testosterone resulted in a marked increase in sexual arousal and improvement in satisfaction with sexual activity.

Failure to ejaculate or difficulty in ejaculation has been reported by several patients receiving Valium or Librium (Hughes, 1964; Munjack, 1979). Munjack (1979) speculates that this effect is likely central rather than peripheral in origin.

EXPERIMENTAL STUDIES

Chetanasilpin and co-workers (1975) examined psychosexual response to erotic stimuli in 10 males after placebo or diazepam (5 mg). Measures of sexual stimulation included changes in blood pressure, heart rate, and respiration rate. Under diazepam, blood pressure was significantly elevated but heart rate and respiration rate were not affected significantly.

EFFECTS ON HORMONES

Arguellis and Rosner (1975) reported that after two weeks of diazepam (10–20 mg) treatment, plasma testosterone levels were significantly elevated in a group of men compared to a nontreated group. No data was presented as to predrug levels or method of analysis.

EFFECTS ON MENSTRUATION

Schwartz and Smith (1963) reported that Librium (20–30 mg) did not affect duration of menstruation in a group of patients (N=35) being treated for infertility. One of the patients did not ovulate prior to drug treatment but after drug treatment ovulation was initiated. Six of the patients eventually became pregnant while on medication.

STUDIES IN ANIMALS

Leavitt (1969) reported that diazepam (2.5 and 5.0 mg/kg) significantly impaired sexual behavior in male rats. At the higher doses, many of the animals were unable to complete testing. At the lower dose, sexual activity was disrupted especially in terms of mounting frequency (mounting without intromission).

Cook *et al.* (1979) reported that chronic treatment with diazepam (50 mg/kg) produced a slight but nonsignificant decrease in testes weight but did reduce the weight of the ventral prostate significantly. Serum testosterone levels were also reduced significantly. Serum LH, FSH, or hypothalamic levels of LH–RH were not affected.

Summary and Conclusions

Despite the widespread use of benzodiazepine there has been relatively little notice of sexually-related side effects of these drugs. When such reports have appeared, they tend to be contradictory. Effects on testosterone levels are also at variance when human and animal studies are compared. At present, the general lack of agreement in effects and the general absence of reference to sexual side effects suggests that these drugs probably do not have any direct effect on sexual arousal, behavior, or function.

References

Ansari, J. M. A. Impotence: Prognosis (a controlled study). *British Journal of Psychiatry*, 1976, *128*, 194–198.

Arguelles, A. E. and Rosner, J. Diazepam and plasma-testosterone levels. *Lancet*, 1975, 2, 607.

Carney, A., Bancroft, J., and Mathews, A. Combination of hormonal and psychological treatment for female sexual unresponsiveness: A comparative study. *British Journal of Psychiatry*, 1978, *132*, 339–346.

Chetanasilpin, P., Tuchinda, P., and Chenpanich, K. Effects of some drugs on psychosexual response in man. *Journal of the Medical Association of Thailand*, 1975, *58*, 509–514.

Cook, P. S., Notelovitz, M., Kalra, P. S., and Kalra, S. P. Effect of diazepam on serum testosterone and the ventral prostate gland in male rats. *Archives of Andrology*, 1979, *3*, 31–35.

Hughes, J. M. Failure to ejaculate with chlordiazepoxide. *American Journal of Psychiatry*, 1964, *121*, 610–611.

Leavitt, F. I. Drug-induced modifications in sexual behavior and open field locomotion of male rats. *Physiology and Behavior*, 1969, *4*, 677–683.

Maneksha, S. and Harry, T. V. A. Lorazepam in sexual disorders. *British Journal of Clinical Practice*, 1975, *29*, 175–176.

Munjack, D. J. Sex and drugs. *Clinical Toxicology*, 1979, *15*, 75–89.

Schwartz, E. D. and Smith, J. J. The effect of chlordiazepoxide on the female reproductive cycle as tested in infertility patients. *Western Journal of Surgery, Obstetrics, and Gynecology*, 1963, *71*, 74–76.

Usdin, G. L. Preliminary report on Librium, a new psychopharmacologic agent. *Journal of the Louisiana State Medical Society*, 1960, *112*, 142–147.

Chapter 8

Cocaine

Cocaine is a CNS stimulant that increases alertness, elevates mood, and produces euphoria. It was isolated from the leaves of the *Erythroxylon coca* tree in the 1860s and around the turn of the century was used as a local anesthetic, but currently has no clinical uses.

Cocaine is a white crystalline powder which is generally taken by sniffing through a straw into the nostrils. Less frequently it is taken by injection. Effects are very similar to those produced by the amphetamines. At low doses (about 20 mg) euphoria, self-confidence, and decreased fatigue are experienced. At higher doses (about 200 mg), euphoria may still be experienced, but other effects such as dizziness, uncontrollable twitching, agitation, and paranoia may occur. Chronic use is accompanied by insomnia, increased sensitivity to noise, agitation, paranoia, confusion, and exhaustion. Tolerance does not occur to the stimulant effects and abstinence is not followed by a withdrawal syndrome.

Like the amphetamines, cocaine inhibits reuptake of norepinephrine into presynaptic terminals thereby increasing and prolonging the amount of NE in the synapse. However, cocaine differs from the amphetamines in having a considerably shorter duration of action (5–15 min) compared to the amphetamines (several hours). This is because cocaine is rapidly metabolized by the liver whereas the amphetamines are not.

Of all the psychoactive drugs whose usage has been linked with sexual arousal, cocaine is the *primus inter pares*. The expression "sex-crazed dope fiend," first arose as a description of the chronic cocaine user (Cohen, 1975; Ellinwood, 1975). "A shot of cocaine," writes Selden (1979), "feels more like an orgasm than anything in the world except an orgasm."

The roots of this link between cocaine and sexual stimulation can be traced back to the time of the Spanish conquistadores when they first encountered the libidinous art of the native Peruvians. To these Spaniards, the "sodomistic, homosexual and bestial perversions" (Bejarno, 1952) portrayed in such pictures had to be due to some unique influence, and the unique influence they felt to be responsible was the natives' use of coca. More than a century later, the behavior depicted in the iconography of the Peruvians was explained as due to cocaine-induced stimulation of the "libido center" (Valdizan, 1915).

Current beliefs concerning cocaine and sex date back to the early 20th century and regard cocaine as a drug that can, and often does, unleash uncontrollable sexual and aggressive impulses—the "sex crazed dope-fiend" stereotype. In part, this caricature may have stemmed from the prescription of some physicians around the turn of the century of cocaine to treat premature ejaculation (Cohen, 1975) and from early newspaper stories attributing sex-related crimes by blacks to their use of cocaine (Helmer, 1975). This caricature still remains. Wilson (1973), for instance, described cocaine as a drug with "the most licentious reputation of any chemical and probably deserves it."

As is typical with other drugs associated with sexual arousal, there is also a considerable literature describing opposite effects. In 1903, in their report to the American Pharmaceutical Association, for instance, Eberle and Gordon took solace in their statement that "one redeeming feature there is: The habitual use of cocaine seems to lessen both sexual desire and ability so there is less danger of its transmission by heredity." Other clinicians also reported diminished sexual arousal and performance associated with chronic cocaine use (Chopra and Chopra, 1930; Gutierrez-Noreiga, 1947).

During the 1920s, some clinicians (e.g., Joel & Frankel, 1924) claimed that excessive use of cocaine could turn a heterosexual into a homosexual and this notion was endorsed by other clinicians and anti-drug propagandists (e.g., Chopra & Chopra, 1930; Wolff, 1932).

Since there is no experimental data with which to assess these claims, the following survey will deal primarily with literary and anecdotal reports, survey studies, and studies in animals.

MALE SEXUALITY

Literary and Anecdotal Reports

In general, literary and anecdotal reports about cocaine and sex distinguish between initial effects and effects experienced after chronic prolonged usage. For example, in his novel *Cocaine*, published in 1921, Pitigrili writes:

> "in the early stages, taking cocaine had resulted in a sensual restlessness, an almost insatiable erotic excitement which two mistresses had not been sufficient to satisfy"

but as usage continued, cocaine

> "had begun to lower the flame of his passions. His sensuality was now a tiny flame on the point of extinction."

Although the Spanish conquerors regarded cocaine as an aphrodisiac, in his description of the Kogi, a tribe in Colombia, Blejer-Prieto (1965) describes an initiation rite in which cocaine is regarded as a sexual substitute:

> "The young man receives the small gourd of lime with which the coca he chews will be mixed, and he is made to understand that the small receptacle represents a woman. The young man is married to this woman during the ceremony, and perforates the gourd in imitation of the ritual deflowering; the small twig with which he does this symbolizes the penis. The introduction of the twig into the small gourd or

receptacle and the gesture of rubbing round the opening are interpreted as the symbolizing of the sexual act, and in their culture this
means that all sexual intercourse is to be abandoned, its only manifestations or expression being the symbolic use of coca."

Philips and Wynne (1974) quote a cocaine user who acknowledged cocaine's reputation as a sexual stimulant, but claimed that
much of its reputation was due to the situation in which it was
used:

"Everybody says that it's an aphrodisiac. Again, I think some people
say it because it's supposed to be. I think that it's just peer group
identification. I remember when I first started doing coke. I remember
everybody would be sitting around saying, "Oh, I just go to get laid."
I said it a couple of times, but I never felt that way. I was more content
to sit there and enjoy it."

These literary and anecdotal reports can thus be recited as
evidence for almost any claim regarding cocaine and sex.

SURVEY STUDIES AND CLINICAL REPORTS

Early clinical reports (e.g., Vervaeck, 1923; Maier, 1926) noted
that while many cocaine users experienced an initial sexual excitement and delayed ejaculation, continued usage resulted in impotence and frigidity.

Summaries of interviews with cocaine users (e.g., Ashley,
1975; Grinspoon & Bakalar, 1976; Spotts & Shontz, 1980) likewise
note initial cocaine-induced sexual stimulation, including reports
of spontaneous erection, prolonged priapism, and multiple
orgasm. Selden (1979) writes that the usual dosage associated with
this effect is about 10–15 mg cocaine hydrochloride. However,
continued usage often results in loss of libido and decreased sexual
performance. Masseur-prostitutes interviewed by Wesson (1982)
considered cocaine to affect sexual performance adversely while
still increasing libido. Some of the adverse effects they report are
clients' inability to achieve erection and delayed time to ejaculation
(although the latter may be considered a positive effect among
clients).

Clinical studies also note that one of the ways cocaine is used is as a topical anesthetic in the areas of the genitals or anus. This acts to prolong sexual activity by lengthening time to ejaculation. In this regard, Gay and Sheppard (1973) report having had to treat several women for "inflamed, raw mucosa of the vaginal vault" who had had sexual partners that had used cocaine in this way.

The most systematic interview studies of cocaine and the association of such drug use with sexuality are those conducted by the Haight-Ashbury Free Medical Clinic (e.g., Gay & Sheppard, 1972; Gay *et al.*, 1982; Newmeyer, 1975). In these studies, previously drug-oriented patients undergoing detoxification have been sampled. When asked which drug they would choose to enhance sex, cocaine was chosen as frequently as alcohol and far less often than marihuana. One possible reason for this bias, however, may have been the much higher cost of cocaine compared to other drugs such as marihuana: "There is little question, but that, were cocaine as cheap and as readily available as marijuana, it would supplant grass as the premium pharmacological adjunct to the erotic practices of our youthful population" (Gay *et al.*, 1977). This opinion is borne out by those asked to rate specific drug effects on sexual functioning. Cocaine was rated as the most effective drug compared to heroin, marihuana, alcohol, barbiturates, and other drugs, in increasing sensuality, likelihood of achieving orgasm, increasing libido, increasing ability to maintain erection, increasing ability to control ejaculation, and increasing sexual fantasy.

In a subsequent study (Gay *et al.*, 1982), 102 "gourmet" respondents from previously sex-oriented groups were surveyed. These were mainly middle class individuals and included heterosexuals and homosexuals. Cocaine was used by more than 50% of the respondents and was rated as third overall (after marihuana and alcohol) as the drug most used "to make sex better." However, when sexual preference was considered, cocaine was chosen equally as often by heterosexual men (but was still third among heterosexual women). Cocaine (along with LSD) was rated fourth (after marihuana, MDA and nitrites) in actually increasing sexual pleasure. Among heterosexual men, however, cocaine was cited as third among the drugs used to increase sexual pleasure (and was cited as third among heterosexual women). Cocaine was also cited as being the most positively enhancing among drugs increasing sexual arousal.

In comparing these results from data from their previous study with detoxification patients, Gay *et al.* (1982) note that cocaine was not as positively rated in the later study. One reason for this discrepancy, they suggest, may have been the increased representation of homosexuals who were much less enthusiastic about cocaine compared to heterosexuals.

Nail and co-workers (1974) interviewed approximately 1,000 navy men who applied for amnesty and help for drug use. Reasons for cocaine use were primarily hedonistic with heightened sexual pleasure being the primary motive for use. The percentage of heavy cocaine users reporting having used cocaine primarily for sexual enhancement was greater than the percentage using any other drug.

Siegel (1977) interviewed 85 "social-recreation cocaine users" whose minimal usage was 1 gram per month. About 13% reported drug-related sexual stimulation during acute usage and 4% reported sexual impotence associated with chronic usage. In a subsequent study, Siegel (1982) inquired into sexual functioning in 32 cocaine users (both male and female) requesting clinical attention. Thirteen of the users reported not engaging in any sexual activity during cocaine use. Twenty of the men reported situational impotence while 4 of the women reported enhanced sexual performance. When the spouses of sexual partners of these users were interviewed, all stated that their partners exhibited sexual disinterest. On the basis of his studies, Siegel (1982) regards the continuing appeal of cocaine as a sexual stimulant despite drug-induced sexual dysfunction and decreased libido or delayed orgasm to be due to nonpsychopharmacological effects.

Jeri and his co-workers (1978a,b) distinguished several phases of cocaine-related effects on sex on the basis of interviews with cocaine users admitted for psychiatric care in Peru. The first phase was cocaine euphoria characterized by intense pleasure and hyper-sexuality (experienced by about 11% of users). Next came a period of cocaine dysphoria consisting of anxiety and sexual indifference. The last phase of cocaine hallucinations was also marked by sexual indifference and impotence.

STUDIES IN ANIMALS

Leavitt (1969) administered cocaine (10, 30 mg/kg, i.p.) to male rats that had had previous sexual experience. Animals were tested with females in estrus. The drug had a biphasic effect on sexual behavior. The lower dose facilitated sexual activity as reflected in significantly lower ejaculation and post-ejaculation latencies, whereas the higher dose increased such latencies. Motor activity was increased at both doses.

EFFECTS ON HORMONES

Surprisingly, few articles could be located in which the effects of cocaine on sex hormones has been reported. In one study (Gordon *et al.*, 1980) rats were injected (i.p.) with about 30 mg/kg cocaine HCl. Control animals were injected with vehicle. Animals were then anesthetized with ether at various times after injection and sacrificed. Animals injected with cocaine had significantly higher testosterone levels at 90 and 120 minutes after injection compared to controls. At 180 minutes after injection, however, testosterone levels in cocaine-treated animals fell significantly below those in control.

Ravitz and Moore (1977) administered cocaine HCl (0, 10, 20, 40 mg/kg) to male rats. Animals were sacrificed 30 minutes later. Cocaine produced a small but dose-related decrease in serum prolactin levels. The decrease was significant only for those receiving the highest dose of drug.

Effects on Reproductive Tissue

In animals, cocaine is distributed to all tissues and, therefore, could have a direct outcome on reproductive tissues. However, few studies have as yet been conducted in this area.

Cocaine has been reported to increase uterine contractions in the rabbit *in vitro* (Daniel & Wolowyk, 1966), but whether levels of cocaine are high enough to do so *in vivo* is not known. Interestingly, the uterus accumulates relatively high levels of cocaine compared to other tissues (Shah *et al.*, 1980).

In small dogs, cocaine did not affect prostate secretion induced by drugs that produce such secretion (Smith & Ilievski, 1969).

Loewe (1938) reported that cocaine had no effect on ejaculation volume associated with death-induced ejaculation in mice, although methamphetamine did increase ejaculation volume.

Summary and Conclusions

Cocaine's reputation as an aphrodisiac has never been disproven, and there is considerable anecdotal and survey data in support of this belief. As with most drugs, effects are dose-related and as dose increases, previous experiences of enhanced libido and sexual performance are reversed. This general pattern is supported by the single study in animals that has been reported. In light of the long interest in cocaine and its colored reputation, one would have expected considerably more information to be available regarding its effects on human and animal sexual behavior and physiology. This is certainly one area of sex-related research that would prove interesting and informative.

References

Ashley, R. *Cocaine.* Warner Books, New York, 1975.

Bejarno, J. Further considerations on the coca habit in Colombia. *Bulletin on Narcotics.* 1952, 4(3), 3–19.

Blejer-Prieto, H. Coca leaf and cocaine addiction—some historical notes. *Canadian Medical Association Journal,* 1965, 93, 700–704.

Burroughs, W. S. *Junkie*. Ace, New York, 1953.

Byck, R. and Van Dyke, C. What are the effects of cocaine in man? NIDA Research Monograph, 1977, *Series 13*, 97–117.

Chopra, R. and Chopra, G. Cocaine habit in India. *Indian Journal of Medical Research*, 1930, *18*, 1013–1046.

Cohen, S. Cocaine. *Journal of the American Medical Association*, 1975, *231*, 74–75.

Crowley, A. *Diary of a Drug Fiend*. William Collins Sons, London, 1922.

Daniel, E. E. and Wolowyk, M. The contractile response of the uterus to cocaine. *Canadian Journal of Physiology and Pharmacology*, 1966, *44*, 721–730.

Eberle, E. G. and Gordon, F. T. Report of Committee on the Acquirement of drug habits. *American Journal of Pharmacology*, 1903, *75*, 474–489.

Ellinwood, E. H. and Rockwell, W. J. K. Effect of drug use on sexual behavior. *Medical Aspects of Human Sexuality*, 1975, *9*, 10–32.

Gay, G. R., Newmeyer, J. A., Elion, R. A., and Wieder, S. The sensuous hippie: Drug/sex practice in the Haight-Ashbury. *Drug Forum*, 1977, *6*(1), 27–47.

Gay, G. R. and Sheppard, C. W. Sex in the "Drug Culture." *Medical Aspects of Human Sexuality*, 1972, *6*(10), 28–50.

Gay, G. R., Newmeyer, J. A., Perry, M., Johnson, G., and Kurland, M. Love and Haight: The sensuous hippie revisited, drug/sex practices in San Francisco, 1980–81. *Journal of Psychoactive Drugs*, 1982, *14*, 111–123.

Gay, G. R. and Sheppard, C. W. Sex-crazed dope fiends—myth or reality? *Drug Forum*, 1973, *2*(2), 225–240.

Goode, E. Marijuana and sex. *Evergreen Review*, 1969, *66*, 19.

Gordon, L. A., Mostofsky, D. I., and Gordon, G. G. Changes in testosterone levels in the rat following intraperitoneal cocaine HCl. *International Journal of Neuroscience*, 1980, *11*, 139–141.

Gottlieb, A. *Sex Drugs and Aphrodisiacs*. High Times, New York, 1974.

Grinspoon, L. and Bakalar, J. B. *Cocaine: A drug and its social evolution*. Basic Books, Inc., New York, 1976.

Gutierez-Noreiga, C. Alteraciones mentales proudecas por a coca. (Mental alterations proceeding from coca). *Revisita de Neuro-Psiquiatria*, 1947, *10*, 145–176.

Hollander, X., Moore, R., and Dunleavy, Y. *The happy hooker*. Dell Publishing Company, New York, 1972.

Helmer, J. *Drugs and Minority Oppression*. New York, Seabury Press, 1975.

Jeri, F. R., Sanchez, C. C., del Pozo, T., Fernandez, M., and Carbajal, C. Further experience with the syndromes produced by coca paste smoking. *Bulletin on Narcotics*, 1978a, *30*(3), 1–11.

Jeri, F. R., Sanchez, C., DelPozo, T., and Fernandez, M. The syndrome of coca paste. *Journal of Psychoactive Drugs*, 1978b, *10*, 361–370.

Joel and Frankel: Der Cocainismus, Berlin, 1924.

Leavitt, F. I. Drug-induced modification in sexual behavior and open field locomotion of male rats. *Physiology and Behavior*, 1969, *4*, 677–683.

Loewe, S. Ejaculation induced by drug action. *Archives Internationales de Pharmacodynamic et de Therapie*, 1938, *60*(1).

Maier, H. W. *Der kokainismus*, Georg Thieme, Lepizig, 1926.

Nail, R. L., Gunderson, E., and Kolb, D. Motives for drug use among light and heavy users. *The Journal of Nervous and Mental Disease*, 1974, *2*, 13–136.

Newmeyer, J. A. *The current status of cocaine use in the San Francisco bay area.* In *Drug abuse.* Marcel Dekker, Inc., New York, 1975.

Philips, J. L. and Wynne, R. D. *A cocaine bibliography—nonannotated.* National Institute on Drug Abuse, Rockville, Md., 1974.

Pitigrilli. (Originally published in 1921). *Cocaine.* Hamlyn Paperbacks. Berkeley, 1974.

Ravitz, A. J. and Moore, K. E. Effects of amphetamine, Methylphenidate and Cocaine on serum prolactin concentrations in the male rat. *Life Sciences,* 1977, *21,* 267–272.

Selden, G. *Aphrodisia.* E. P. Dutton, New York, 1979.

Shah, N. S., May, D. A., and Yates, J. D. Disposition of levo—(H) cocaine in pregnant and nonpregnant mice. *Toxicology and Applied Pharmacology,* 1980, *53,* 279–284.

Siegel, R. K. *Cocaine: Recreational Use and Intoxication.* In: Petersen, R. C. and Stillman, R. C. (eds.), *Cocaine, National Institute on Drug Abuse,* Rockville, Md., 1977, pp. 119–136.

Siegel, R. K. Cocaine and sexual dysfunction: The curse of mama coca. *Journal of Psychoactive Drugs,* 1982, *14,* 71–74.

Smith, E. R. and Ilievski, V. The stimulation of canine prostatic secretion by substances. *Proceedings of the Society for Experimental Biology and Medicine,* 1969, *130*(2), 667–671.

Spotts, J. V. and Shontz, F. C. *Cocaine users. A representative case approach.* New York: Free Press, 1980.

Valdizan, H. La Alienacion mental entre los primitivos Peruanos. Lima, Peru: Pacific Press, 1915.

Vervaeck, L. Quelques aspects medicaux et psychologiques de la cocaineomanie. *LaScalpel,* 1923, *76,* 744.

Wesson, D. R. Cocaine use by masseuses. *Journal of Psychoactive Drugs,* 1980, *14,* 75–76.

Wesson, D. R. and Smith, D. E. Cocaine: Its use for central nervous system stimulation including recreational and medical uses. *NIDA Research Monograph No. 13,* 1977.

Wilson, R. A. *Sex and drugs.* Playboy Press, Chicago, 1973.

Wolff, P. Drug addiction—a worldwide problem. *Journal of the American Medical Association,* 1932, 175–184.

Chapter 9

Coffee

Caffeine, the main psychoactive ingredient in coffee, is among the most widely used stimulants in the world. Although consumed mainly in the form of coffee, it is also found in cola drinks, chocolate, cocoa, and tea. An average cup of coffee contains about 100–150 mg of caffeine. Other beverages contain considerably less.

At low doses (150 mg), caffeine produces increased alertness, decreased fatigue, and mood elevation. Nervousness and insomnia are also experienced by those who use it infrequently. At larger doses (about 400 mg) nervousness, irritability, insomnia, irregular heart beat, and increased blood pressure occur. Tolerance develops to the stimulant effects and physical dependence also occurs. Withdrawal is associated with headache, lethargy, and nausea.

The primary site of action in the brain is the cortex followed by the brain stem. The mechanism of action appears to involve intracellular functioning such as increased permeability of nerve fibers to calcium, accumulation of intracellular "messengers" such as cyclic AMP, which acts to potentiate effects of hormones, and blockade of receptors for adenosine, which may affect adrenergic neurotransmission.

Although coffee is one of the most widely used substances, there is virtually no information concerning its effects on sexual activity or performance. There are, however, a number of anecdotal remarks worth noting. The first comes from a thesis written in 1695 at the École de Medicine in Paris, in which the author comments that daily use of coffee decreases sexual drive (quoted by Davenport, 1873). There is also a comment by a "celebrated" surgeon of past centuries that "any man that drinks coffee and soda water, and smokes cigars, may lie with my wife" (quoted by Davenport, 1873).

Lewin (1964) comments that "it has frequently been stated that the drinking of coffee diminishes sexual excitability and gives rise to sterility." Lewin also relates several amusing anecdotes in this regard. According to one such anecdote, a Sultan drank so much coffee he lost interest in his wife. Later on, when he happened to see a stallion being castrated, he said that giving the animal coffee would achieve the same purpose. Another anecdote quoted by Lewin concerns Princess Charlotte, mother of King Philip II of Orleans, who wrote to her sisters: "Coffee is not so necessary for Protestant ministers as for Catholic priests, who are not allowed to marry and must remain chaste."

EFFECTS IN ANIMALS

In an early study, Loewe (1938) evaluated the effects of caffeine on death-induced ejaculation in mice. Under such conditions, caffeine had no effect, although other stimulants did induce ejaculation.

Zimbardo and Barry (1958) injected (i.p.) male rats with 20 mg/kg caffeine. Caffeine decreased latency to mount, copulate, and ejaculate. Similar observations have also been reported by Soulairac and Coppin-Monthillaud (1951).

Soulairac and Soulairac (1978) reported that injection of caffeine restored sexual behavior in male rats that had been unresponsive to females following decortication (of the males). Prior to decortication pre-copulatory latency was 8.6 minutes. After decortication, it was 49.7 minutes. After caffeine, latency was 2.2 minutes for decorticated males.

EFFECTS ON SPERM

Several studies have noted that caffeine increases sperm motility. Schoenfeld *et al.* (1973) incubated human semen samples with caffeine. Caffeine produced an increase in the number of motile sperm, from 16% to 27% in one sample and 35% to 52% in another, improved their activity, and increased their longevity. Similar results were reported by Haesungcharern and Chulavatnatol (1973), Bunge (1973), Barkay *et al.* (1977), and Harrison (1978).

Harrison (1978) assessed the rate of caffeine-stimulated sperm activity on artificial insemination. Most of the sperm samples had very low motility. Although sperm motility was increased, addition of caffeine to the samples did not increase pregnancy rate among these infertile females.

SUMMARY AND CONCLUSIONS

Very little is known about the effects of caffeine on sexual arousal or performance despite the ubiquity of this substance. This would certainly appear to be an area where additional information would be welcome.

References

Barkay, J., Zuckerman, H., Sklan, D., Shmuel, G. Effect of caffeine on increasing the motility of frozen human sperm. *Fertility and Sterility*, 1977, *28*, 175.

Bunge, R. G. Caffeine-stimulation of ejaculated human spermatozoa. *Urology, University of Iowa Hospitals*, 1973, *1*, 371.

Davenport, J. Aphrodisiacs and love stimulants. 1873, Repr. Lyle Stuart, New York, 1966.

Haesungcharern, A. and Chulavatnatol, M. Stimulation of human spermatozoal motility by caffeine. *Fertility and Sterility*, 1973, *24*, 662.

Harrison, R. F. Insemination of husband's semen with and without the addition of caffeine. *Fertility and Sterility*, 1978, *29*, 532.

Lewin, L. *Phantastica*, E. P. Dutton, New York, 1964.

Loewe, S. Ejaculation induced by drug action. *Archives Internationales de Pharmacodynamic et de Therapie*, 1938, *60*, 37.

Schoenfeld, C., Amelar, R. D., and Dubin, L. Stimulation of ejaculated human spermatozoa by caffeine. A Preliminary Report. *Fertility and Sterility*, 1973, *24*, 772.

Soulairac, A. and Coppin-Monthillaud, M. Effects of caffeine and chlorpromazine on the sexual behavior of male rats. *Journal of Physiology*, 1951, *43*, 869.

Soulairac, A. and Soulairac, M. Relationship between the nervous and endocrine regulation of sexual behavior in male rats. *Psychoneuroendocrinology*, 1978, *3*, 17–29.

Zimbardo, P. G. and Barry, H. Effects of caffeine and chlorpromazine on the sexual behavior of male rats. *Science*, 1958, *127*, 84–85.

Chapter 10

Hallucinogens

Hallucinogens are drugs that can produce illusions—distorted perceptions of visual, auditory, tactile, gustatory, and kinesthetic sensory information. These drugs can also produce true hallucinations—experiences which do not conform to physical reality such as seeing or hearing people or objects that do not exist. Yet another perceptual distortion is synthesia—sensation in one sensory mode being perceived in another, e.g., hearing colors, seeing sounds. In addition to these effects, they also produce euphoria, depression, or anxiety.

Most hallucinogens used today are synthetic substances that resemble naturally occurring substances. While there are many different kinds of hallucinogens, the two such compounds for which there is the most information concerning effects on sexuality are LSD and PCP and therefore only these two drugs will be discussed here.

LSD

LSD (lysergic acid diethylamide) was synthesized in 1938 and occurs naturally in ergot, a fungus that grows on rye and other grains. LSD is the most potent of all the hallucinogens. A minimal effective dose is about 50–100 micrograms. It is usually taken orally, but is sometimes inhaled or injected.

Effects vary widely and include visual and auditory hallucinations, distortions of body image and time, alterations of thought and mood, and deep introspection.

Adverse reactions ("bad trips") include acute paranoia, confusion, disorientation, and loss of reality. Spontaneous recurrence of brief experiences ("flashbacks") sometimes also occur long after drug use has been discontinued.

The mechanism of action for LSD is believed to be due to its structural resemblance to serotonin.

During the 1960s, LSD was regarded as the prototype psychedelic aphrodisiac, a drug endowed with a potpourri of sexual effects ranging from inducement of orgasms in primarily non-orgasmic users, to a cure for homosexuality (Freedman, 1976). Former head of the Bureau of Narcotics, Henry J. Anslinger (1966), commented, for example, that "as to LSD. . . The principal side effect of taking it is pregnancy . . . we should call LSD 'Let's Start Degeneracy'."

Several anecdotal comments quoted by Gay and Sheppard (1973) are also supportive of LSD's enhancement of sexual experience:

> "To make love on acid is to make perfect love and gain protoplasmic unity." "When I come (on LSD) my whole soul and body seem to fuse (with my partner)."

Leary (1968) likewise emphasized the enhancement of the sensual side of sexual activity associated with LSD:

> ". . . The LSD experience is . . . all lovemaking. You make love with candlelight, with sound waves from a record player, with the trees. . . Compared with sex under LSD, the way you've been making love— no matter how ecstatic the pleasure you think you get from it—is like making love to a department store window dummy."

Other reports claimed that LSD use could result in impotence (Dahlberg, 1971):

> "One mature man of undoubted virility became impotent with his newly married wife following one horrendous LSD trip. Under the

influence of the drug, he hallucinated her as a shark and thereafter this image was repeated whenever he attempted intercourse with her."

Still other reports were considerably more circumspect, stressing the substitution of drug use for sexual contact (Freedman, 1976):

"One man we heard of who claimed phenomenal sexual powers while under the influence of drugs (such as LSD) was observed during his entire trip crouched in a corner."

Sexual Effects

Alpert (1969) described one of his patients, a 38-year-old male who "had been acting out homosexual behavior since the age of fifteen." After several treatments with LSD (200 µg), the man overcame his panic concerning sexual activity with women and engaged in sexual intercourse. "One year later: Our subect has now been living with a woman for eight months. They have been having intercourse every night, except during her periods. He has had two homosexual experiences in that time, and he sought these, he said, mostly to find out 'where he was at' and whether the changes were real."

Gay and Sheppard (1973) reported that 44 of the 48 respondents interviewed by them at the Haight Ashbury Free Medical Clinic expressed the opinion that LSD did not involve libido, but did rate it as enhancing sexual pleasure. Gay and Sheppard (1973) attributed any positive affect on this regard to the "empathy which exists between partners, and to an appropriate setting in which the drug is taken."

In their second study, Gay and co-workers (1977) reported that LSD was rated third to marihuana and cocaine among drugs specifically taken "to make sex better." However, in most cases, LSD was not taken specifically for possible sexual effects.

In rating a number of drugs as to sexual functioning, LSD, along with marihuana and mescaline, was rated as second to cocaine in regard to improvement of sexual functioning. LSD's highest ratings came in response to "ability to have sexual fantasies," and "affecting pleasure associated with touching and being touched." In terms of performance, however, LSD was rated very poorly in terms of achieving and maintaining erection and controlling ejaculation.

In their third study of nonpatient, "privileged middle class" heterosexual and homosexual drug users (Gay *et al.*, 1982), LSD was cited by over one-third of the respondents as a drug taken "to make sex better." The group which rated it highest in this regard was homosexual men who ranked it second to nitrites for enhancing sex. LSD was also rated overall by these respondents as equal to cocaine in increasing sexual pleasure.

Studies in Animals

Male Animals

Bignami (1966) reported that male rats injected with 0.01 and 0.02 mg/kg LSD had lower intromission intervals. Intromission frequency was also increased in animals given 0.02 mg/kg. Post ejaculatory interval was also increased in animals at higher doses (0.2 mg/kg). At the highest dose (1 mg/kg) animals were sedated.

Gillett (1960) administered (i.p.) 130 or 200 μg/kg to sexually experienced male rats. Females were brought into heat by estrogen and progesterone and males were tested after adaptation to the apparatus. Animals injected with LSD engaged in fewer copulations prior to ejaculation. In some instances, however, motor disturbance was so great the copulation was not possible.

Malmnas (1973) administered (s.c.) LSD to castrated male rats given testosterone. A dose of 10 μg/kg did not affect copulatory behavior. Higher doses (30 μg/kg and 100 μg/kg) inhibited copulatory activity. At the 100 μg/kg dose, general activity appeared to be affected.

Female Animals

Eliasson and Meyerson (1976, 1977) and Sietnieks and Meyerson (1980) reported that LSD inhibited estrogen and progesterone induced lordosis in female rats and that this effect was dose-related. Maximal inhibition following LSD (50 µg/kg, i.p.) occurred at 10 minutes after injection. Recovery occurred by three hours after injection (Sietnieks & Meyerson, 1980).

In an earlier study, however, Everitt and co-workers (1974) observed a facilitation of lordosis response by lower doses of LSD (5–20 µg/kg) when lordosis was induced by estrogen only. A higher dose of LSD (40 µg/kg) had no effect. Sietnieks and Meyerson (1980) likewise noted that high doses of LSD (100 µg/kg) had no effect on lordosis when induced by estrogen alone.

PCP

PCP (phencyclidine) was synthesized in 1957 as an anesthetic but was withdrawn due to its hallucinatory effects. It is generally taken orally, but sometimes it is also sprinkled on tobacco or marihuana cigarettes and then smoked, or injected.

Effects vary widely and include hallucinations, distortions of sensory information, euphoria, and impairment of thought processes. At low doses (about 5–10 mg) there is a sense of euphoria and weightlessness. At higher doses (about 20 mg), hallucinogenic and stimulant effects occur along with distortion of body image.

Adverse effects include vomiting, depression, disorientation, agitation, panic, and paranoia after low doses. After higher doses, additional adverse effects include difficulty in moving and thinking. As in the case of LSD, "flashbacks" sometimes also occur.

The mechanism of action is unknown. Structurally, PCP resembles both norepinephrine and serotonin and effects may be due to mimicry of their effects. Experimental studies have also shown it to inhibit reuptake of norepinephrine and acetylcholinesterase activity.

Sexual Effects

Gay and co-workers (1977) reported that PCP was rarely used "to make sex better" by the 95 patients they interviewed at the Haight-Ashbury Free Medical Clinic. Furthermore, few of these respondents stated that they engaged in sex while under the influence of the drug. PCP was rated at the bottom of a list of drugs as stimulating libido and was also rated poorly in terms of enhancing sexual performance. In this regard, the authors comment that "overdose (of PCP) is common among the unsophisticated and the drug glutton may create bizarre and ineffectual sexual experience" (p. 38).

In their subsequent study of nonpatient "gourmet" drug users, Gay and co-workers (1982) likewise noted that PCP was cited as last in a list of drugs used "to make sex better." PCP was likewise rated as last among drugs that increased sexual pleasure. These opinions were general among both men and women and among heterosexuals, homosexuals, and bisexuals.

Smith and co-workers (1980) interviewed 20 PCP users who sought medical assistance at the Haight-Ashbury Free Medical Clinic. When used primarily to affect sexual functioning, the drug was primarily smoked, as opposed to swallowing or injecting. When used sporadically and at low doses, effects on sexuality were regarded as being enhanced in terms of disinhibition and attitude perception rather than increased libido. Erection or ejaculatory failure were not encountered with low doses. With chemic use or after higher doses, decreased libido and erectile or ejaculatory impairment did occur.

Graeven and co-workers (1981) surveyed 200 PCP "street users" who were not in treatment. Users were divided into "heavy chronic" (3 or more times a week), "light chronic" (1 or 2 times a week), and "recreational" users (less than 1 or 2 times a week). Recreational users stated that before using PCP, they felt more "sexual" than heavy chronic users. However, while under the influence of the drug, recreational users rated themselves as fully less "sexual" than heavy chronic users.

Effects on Hormones

Singh and co-workers (1983) injected (i.p.) male rats with PCP (10 and 20 mg/kg) and sacrificed animals at 0, 1, 2, and 4 hours after injection.

There were no effects on testosterone levels at 1 hour after injection, but at 2 and 4 hours testosterone levels were significantly decreased, although these decreases were not dose-related.

LH hormone levels were also decreased at 2 hour post-injection, but not at 1 or 4 hours.

Harclerode and co-workers (1982) likewise reported that PCP decreased serum LH levels in rats about 3 hours after injection.

References

Alpert, R. Drugs and sexual behavior. *Journal of Sex Research*, 1969, 5, 50–56.

Anslinger, H. J. Playboy interview. *Playboy*, 1966, September, 100.

Bignami, G. Pharmacologic influences on mating behavior in the male rat. *Psychopharmacologia*, 1966, 10, 44–58.

Dahlberg, C. C. Sexual behavior in the drug culture. *Medical Aspects of Human Sexuality*, 1971, 5, 64–71.

Eliasson, M. and Meyerson, B. J. Comparison of the action of lysergic acid diethylamide and apomorphine on the copulatory response in the female rat. *Psychopharmacology*, 1976, 49, 301.

Eliasson, M. and Meyerson, B. J. The effects of lysergic acid diethylamide on copulatory behavior in the female rat. *Neuropharmacology*, 1977, 16, 37.

Everitt, B. J., Fuxe, K., and Hokfeldt, T. Inhibitory role of dopamine and 5-hydroxytryptamine in the sexual behavior of female rats. *European Journal of Pharmacology*, 1974, 29, 187.

Freedman, A. M. Drugs and sexual behavior. In *The sexual experience* Sadock, B. J. & Kaplan, H. I. (eds.), Williams and Wilkins, N.Y., 1976, 328–334.

Gay, G. R., Newmeyer, J. A., Perry, M., Johnson, G., and Kurland, M. Love and Haight. The sensuous hippie revisited. Drug/sex practices in San Francisco, 1980–1981. *Journal of Psychoactive Drugs*, 1982, 14, 111–123.

Gay, G. R., Newmeyer, J. A., Elion, R. A., and Wieder, S. The sensuous hippie: Drug/sex practices in the Haight-Ashbury. *Drug Forum*, 1977, 6, 27–47.

Gay, G. R. and Sheppard, C. W. Sex-crazed dope fiends—myth or reality? *Drug Forum*, 1973, 2, 125–140.

Gillett, E. Effects of Chlorpromazine and D-lysergic acid diethylamide on Sex Behavior of Male Rats. *Proceedings of the Society of Experimental Biology and Medicine*, 1960, 103, 392–394.

Graeven, D. B., Sharp, J. G., and Glatt, S. Acute effects of phencyclidine (PCP) on chronic and recreational users. *American Journal of Drug and Alcohol Abuse*, 1981, 8, 39–50.

Harclerode, J. E., Smith, R. S., and Berger, V. E. Marijuana and phencyclidine and their effect through the CNS on the reproductive system. *Archives of Andrology*, 1982, 9, 1.

Leary, T. *The politics of ecstacy*. G. Putnam, New York, 1968.

Malmnas, C. O. Effect of LSD-25, cloridine, and apomorphene on copulatory behavior in the male rat. *Acta Physiologica Scandinavica*, 1973, (Supplement), 96–116.

Sietnieks, A. and Meyerson, B. J. Enhancement by progesterone of lysergic acid diethylamide inhibition of the copulatory response in the female rat. *European Journal of Pharmacology*, 1980, *63*, 57–64.

Singh, H. H., Mathura, C. B., and Brown, R. J. Phencyclidine (PCP): Effects on serum testosterone and luteinizing hormone concentrations in rats. *Research Communications in Substances of Abuse*, 1983, *4*, 193.

Smith, D. E., Smith, N., Buxton, M. E., and Moser, C. PCP and sexual dysfunction. *Journal of Psychedelic Drugs*, 1980, *12*, 3–4.

Chapter 11

Marihuana

Marihuana is a crude preparation made from the leaves or fruiting tops of *Cannabis sativa.* The principal psychoactive ingredient in marihuana, 1-delta-9-tetrahydrocannabinol (Δ^9-THC), was identified and synthesized in the 1960s.

Marihuana is primarily smoked, but occasionally is also baked into food and eaten. When smoked, only about 50–75 percent of the main active ingredient is absorbed. The smallest amount of delta-9-THC that will produce psychoactive effects in humans is about 5 mg. At this dose, effects include euphoria, relaxation, reduction in attention, impaired memory, and distortions of time, space, and body image. Adverse effects include anxiety, panic, and sometimes paranoia. At higher doses (15 mg) effects noted at lower doses are intensified, and hallucinations and synesthesia may occur. Adverse effects include depersonalization, confused thinking, agitation, and paranoia along with cardiovascular and respiratory problems.

Marihuana is primarily metabolized by the liver but some metabolism occurs in the lungs as well when the drug is taken in by smoking. Some of the metabolites are also active. The drug is taken into the blood very rapidly when smoked and is absorbed into various bodily tissues, especially those with high lipid content. The

119

drug is stored in fatty tissue and is slowly released back into the blood. Due to this storage and slow release mechanisms, cannabinoids can be detected in the body as long as 7 days after the last usage. Elimination from the body occurs primarily via feces but some is also excreted in the urine.

Tolerance may develop to some of the effects of marihuana. Withdrawal tends to be relatively mild and includes sleep disturbances, headache, and weight loss.

The mechanism(s) whereby marihuana produces its effects is (are) unknown. The drug has been found to affect aminergic and cholinergic transmitter function, and produces changes in cell membranes and changes in ultrastructures in neurons.

MALE SEXUALITY

Anecdotal/Literary Evidence

Marihuana has a long historical association with sex, but like alcohol, it has been both praised and criticized for its effects on libido and function.

Also, as in the case of alcohol, this contradiction arises out of an absence of factual information concerning the drug, a contradiction which is still evident today for the same reason. For the most part, the only sources of information concerning marihuana's link with sex are old anecdotes and literary references such as the *Arabian Nights*.

Among the ancient medical authorities, Dioscorides (*Materia Medica* 3.165) advised using the juice of the marihuana seed for treating a tired libido whereas Galen (*De Facultatibus Alimentorum* 100.49) and Pliny (*Natural History* 20.97) were of the opinion that eating too many marihuana seeds could bring on impotence.

During the Middle Ages marihuana's alleged usefulness as an aphrodisiac was especially singled out by demonologists in their frequent crusades against witchcraft. In 1615, for example, Giovanni De Ninault, a well-known witch hunter of his era, wrote that marihuana was a main constituent in the ointments and unguents resorted to during the Witches' Sabbath for the express purpose of bringing on the intoxication, the aphrodisia, and the orgies for which the Black Mass was infamous.

Garcia da Orta, whose *Colloquies on the Simples and Drugs of India* was one of the most widely read medical texts of the late Middle Ages (Abel, 1980b), listed aphrodisia as a major effect of marihuana usage. As a result, medical teaching passed on the connection between marihuana and sexual arousal for generations without a second thought.

Folklorists have also ample evidence of marihuana's connection with sex. A love poem of bygone years in England (Abel, 1980b) states:

Aneve last Midsummer no sleep I sought,
But to the field a bag of hemp-seed brought;
I scatter'd round the seed on ev'ry side,
And three times, in a trembling accent, cried
This hemp-seed with my virgin hand I sow
Who shall my true love be, the crop shall mow.

While hemp seed is not cited as having aphrodisiac effects in this poem, its connection with love and marriage was not lost sight of by others who did see such a connection.

As early as 1853, the *United States Dispensatory* listed aphrodisia among marihuana's pharmacological actions and this effect continued to be included in many following editions.

Even earlier, in 1850, American authors such as Frederick Hollick were touting hashish as a cure-all for impotence. Hollick claimed that his research had shown him that hashish was the main ingredient in all known aphrodisiacs and he recommended it enthusiastically to readers of his *Marriage Guide*.

In 1869, Louisa May Alcott, author of *Little Women* and many other popular stories, also told her readers that hashish was an aphrodisiac. In her story, *Perilous Play*, Rose exclaims after kissing a man, "Oh what am I doing? I am mad, for I, too, have taken hashish."

In the Arab countries hashish was often credited with arousing the libido. An ancient Arab poem, for example, tells about the exploits of Abdu'l Haylukh who deflowered 80 virgins in a single night after he smoked hashish.

A story from the Arabian Nights that dates back to the 15th century tells about a girl who fell asleep after eating hashish. So soundly did she sleep, she was believed to have died and she was buried. After the mistake was discovered, the girl was exhumed and the fresh air revived her. Although still under the influence of the drug, the only lingering effects that were noticeable were "her strong appetite for love and food" (Ley, 1843).

Marihuana has long been associated with the Tantric religion in India (Aldrich, 1977) in which religious sex acts under the influence of marihuana are performed as a consecration to the goddess Kali. Marihuana has also been regarded as an aphrodisiac by both the Ayurveda and Unani Tibbi systems of medicine in that country for over a 1,000 years (Dwarakanath, 1965). The Indian Hemp Drugs Commission, on the other hand, remarked on the use of the drug "by ascetics in this country with the ostensible object of destroying sexual appetite" (Indian Hemp Drugs Commission Report).

During the 1930s when marihuana hysteria began sweeping parts of the United States, the sexual promiscuity theme was widely disseminated. In *Here's To Crime*, for example, author Courtney R. Cooper wrote that "the use of marihuana has spread within the last few years so rapidly as to constitute a menace which should receive the attention of every thinking parent in America" (Cooper, 1937). Among the evil effects of the drug was sexual promiscuity and Cooper described one related incident in which a girl smoked marihuana and then suddenly wanted to dance.

> "Immediately everyone wanted to dance. The movements were of sensuosity. After a time, girls began to pull off their clothes. Men weaved naked over them, soon the entire room was one of the wildest sexuality. Ordinary intercourse and several forms of perversion were going on at once, girl to girl, man to man, woman to woman."

Several years later, another writer wrote as if there were no longer any doubt that "marihuana can be a strong aphrodisiac, and for its users there is usually no such thing as normal sex relations" (Wilson, 1949).

Although there has been a sustained interest in marihuana's alleged aphrodisiac attributes, there is very little evidence either to substantiate or refute the drug's supposed effects on the libido.

In recent years there have been several survey studies of marihuana and sex but no epidemiological or clinical studies have been conducted similar to those conducted with respect to alcohol (Abel, 1980) and there have been no laboratory studies of marihuana's effects on sexual arousal, although the technology for such studies is available and has been used to study alcohol and sexual arousal (Wilson, 1976a,b; Wilson, 1976).

In place of direct studies of marihuana's effects on human sexuality, the main thrust of research efforts to date in this area have been concerned with marihuana's effects on sex steroids and sperm. Interestingly, there has been only one study of marihuana's affects on ovulation and sex steroids in women (Kolodny *et al.*, 1979).

SURVEY STUDIES

Several attempts have been made to examine marihuana's effects on sex by means of questionnaires. In general, these studies support the belief that marihuana is associated with increased sexual behavior and enhances sexual enjoyment.

Goode (1972) reported that frequent usage of marihuana was positively correlated with premarital sex and with increasing numbers of different sex partners. In addition, the earlier the experimentation with marihuana, the earlier the initiation into sex.

Almost identical conclusions were drawn by Hochman and Brill (1973) from their survey study of marihuana usage and sexual behavior. In addition, they noted that marihuana usage was not related to homosexual experiences, marriage rate, divorce rate, number of extramarital affairs, pregnancy, or miscarriages.

Whether use of marihuana leads to increased sexual behavior or vice versa cannot be determined from such studies. Nor is it possible to determine if both increased marihuana usage and increased sexual behavior are both the result of a liberal sociocultural background which either encourages or does not discourage such behavior. Whereas there is an association between marihuana and sex in these and other studies, this association may not be unique but merely a reflection of the increased usage of drugs in general. Those who are most willing to experiment with drugs may also be willing to experiment with sex.

One interesting finding that arose out of Koff's survey of sex and marihuana use by college undergraduates (N=345) was that marihuana was perceived as increasing "sexual desire" for women more than for men (Koff, 1974). However, more men than women felt that marihuana enhanced their sexual pleasure. The results are presented in Table 4.

There was also an indication of a dose-response effect in this study. When amount of marihuana usage was taken into account, 50.5% of the men said libido was increased by smoking one marihuana cigarette or less, whereas smoking two or more marihuana cigarettes was associated with only a 34.5% increase in libido. The comparable estimates among women were 70.9% and 49.5% respectively.

In their study of reasons for using marihuana, Fisher and Steckler (1974) found that perceived sexual pleasure also varied

TABLE 4.   Effects of Marihuana Use on Sexual Desire and Enjoyment by College Students[a]

	Men	Women
Sexual desire		
Increased	39.1%	57.8%
Decreased	10.9%	4.8%
No change	50.0%	37.4%
Sexual enjoyment		
Increased	59.8%	42.9%
Decreased	6.5%	6.5%
No change	34.7%	50.6%

[a]Data from Koff (1974).

with amount of marihuana use. Increased "sexual pleasure" was attributed to marihuana use by only 25% of past marihuana users, by 34% of the "occasional" users, by 58% of the "regular" users, and by 70% of the "daily" users.

Marihuana was cited as the drug which most enhanced sexual pleasure by 50 patients who were interviewed at the Haight-Ashbury Free Medical Clinic by Gay and Sheppard (1973). Among the other drugs used by these respondents were alcohol, barbiturates, amphetamines, cocaine, amyl nitrate, psychedelics, and heroin.

In a second study of patients at this same clinic (Gay *et al.*, 1977), marihuana was cited as being used "a few times a week or as often to make sex better" and in response to the question: "If you were going to use a drug tonight or a combination of drugs, which would you choose?" most respondents chose marihuana first, followed in order by heroin, cocaine, and psychedelics. Alcohol was chosen last.

MECHANISMS

Several attempts have been made to explain the alleged effects of marihuana on human sexuality. Bloomquist (1968) contended that it was only a coincidence: "The age span 14–25 needs no aphrodisiac to stimulate either interest or capacity to perform. If young men have the sex act in mind when they use the drug, they will probably move toward a selected partner."

Another commonly offered explanation is set and setting. One of the female respondents questioned by Koff (1974), for instance, had this opinion:

> "Marihuana itself does not in any way increase sexual desire. It is merely the atmosphere (i.e., setting) in which the drug is used, combined with . . . a darkened room with candlelight, incense burning possibly, often just the two alone, which actually promotes sexual desire."

Yet another explanation is that of lowering of inhibitions. "One joint of grass may lower inhibitions and make an individual more open to experimenting with an exotic sexual technique," write Gay and colleagues.

In summary, marihuana is associated with increased sexual activity and enjoyment for many people. This increased sexual activity, however, does not appear to be specifically due to use of marihuana but rather may reflect a sensation-seeking life-style, and drug use and sex are part of such a life-style (Kaestner *et al.*, 1977; Khavari *et al.*, 1977).

Although it is only a general impression, marihuana does appear to enhance sexual enjoyment for many of its users. This effect is dose-dependent, however. One "joint" enhances sex; more than one begins to have a negative affect. Generally, "set" and "setting" assume greater importance, the lower the potency. With increasing potency or frequency of use, pharmacological effects assume greater importance, and "set" and "setting" are less influential in terms of drug responsiveness.

There have also been numerous attempts to account for the reports of enhanced sexual enjoyment in terms of marihuana-related perceptual changes. Specifically, the perceived slowing down of time may create the impression of prolonged sexual involvement and orgasm (Tart, 1971; Traub, 1977). Tactual sensitivity may also be affected (Tart, 1971; Traub, 1977). Without physiological measurements of sexual arousal, however, it is not possible to relate these perceptual effects to actual bodily changes. Until relevant physiological assessments are forthcoming, evaluation of marihuana's potential to increase sexual arousal, function, or enjoyment will remain speculative.

Effects in Animals

Several studies have examined the effects of cannabinoid compounds on sexual behavior in animals. Such studies, of course, eliminate variables such as "set" and "setting" which may influence sexual behavior in humans. However, these studies in animals are not without their own methodological problems.

In animals such as the rat and mouse, two species whose sexual behavior has been studied in depth and whose sexual behavior in response to drugs such as marihuana has also been examined, sexual behavior is very stereotyped so that variations in this behavioral pattern can be easily recognized and recorded.

Sexual behavior for the male begins with approaching and sniffing the female. The female genitalia are then sniffed and possibly licked. If the female is not in estrus, she will be resistant to any efforts on the part of the male to mount her. If she is in estrus, she may scamper away at the male's initial approach but will then wait for the male to approach once more. The male will again sniff and lick and then attempt to mount. As he does so, the female adopts the lordosis position which involves an arching of the back and the raising and exposing of the genitalia with the tail to one side. The male inserts his penis and begins copulatory movements ("intromissions") which may or may not result in ejaculation. Ejaculation in the rat rarely occurs after the first intromission. After each intromission, the male leaps backwards and sits on his haunches and licks his penis. Each intromission sequence lasts only about five seconds or less and the inter-intromission period may also last only a few seconds or up to several minutes. The sequence is repeated several times, sometimes taking over an hour or more, until ejaculation finally occurs. Male sexual behavior is scored with respect to latency to mount, latency to intromit, and latency to ejaculate.

The female's sexual behavior consists primarily of whether or not she is sexually receptive to the male as reflected in lordosis. The female rat and mouse enter estrus about once every four or five days so that it is important to test females for sexual receptivity during this period. It is also important for the female to be in estrus if any valid test of male sexual behavior is to be made, since male sexual behavior is dependent to an important extent on the receptivity of the female. (One means of bringing female rats or mice into estrus is by injecting them with two injections of estradiol benzoate 24 hours apart, followed 24 hours after the second injection with an injection of progesterone.)

A summary of the effects of cannabinoids on male sexual behavior in animals is presented in Table 5. As indicated by the table, in most studies drug administration has resulted in an inhibition of male sexual activity. However, in most instances, no systematic studies of associated changes in locomotor activity were conducted so that it is not possible to determine if the effects on sexual behavior were specific or were symptomatic of a general decrease in motor activity or general malaise.

Another important consideration is that in several of these studies the estrus cycle of the stimulus female was unknown so that "inhibition" of sexual behavior may have been the result of an unreceptive female.

The most thorough studies of the effects of cannabinoids on male sexual behavior in animals are those conducted by Dalterio and her co-workers (1978; 1980). Although these studies also failed to conduct systematic studies of general motor activity, they do suggest a general impairment of male sexual behavior in mice following drug treatment. Moreover, studies from Dalterio's group also indicate that continued drug treatment affects male sexual behavior to a greater degree than acute treatment. When mice were intubated with Δ^9-THC three times a week for 2.5 weeks, latency to mount increased significantly whereas latency to mount for control animals decreased. Similarly, the number of mounts decreased after repeated drug administration whereas the number of mounts per test session increased for control animals. Continued drug administration for 6 weeks did not further exacerbate these effects; in fact, some degree of tolerance may have occurred since the number of mounts increased over the 2.5 week period (Dalterio, 1980).

The relevance of these animal studies overall to humans, however, is still unsettled. In addition to the much higher dosage levels used in animal studies compared to those consumed by humans, there is the general discrepancy betweeen the effects of cannabinoids on consummatory behaviors in animals and humans. For example, whereas cannabinoids tend to increase consummatory behaviors such as eating in humans, the opposite occurs in

TABLE 5. Effects of Cannabinoid Compounds on Male Sexual Behavior in Animals

Species	Compound & dose	Sexual behavior	Reference
Rat	Δ^9-THC (2 or 3 mg/kg, i.p.)	↓ (Latency to mount) ↓ (Latency to ejaculate)	Merari (1973)
Rat	Hashish resin (8 or 16 mg/kg, Δ^9-THC)	↓ (Copulatory activity—at least 1 intromission)	Corcoran *et al.* (1974)
Rat	Δ^9-THC (0.25 mg/kg, i.p.)	↓ (Competition for females)	Uyeno (1976)
Mouse	Cannabis tincture (12.5 or 25 mg/kg, i.p.)	↓ (Mounting)	Cutler *et al.* (1975)
Mouse	Δ^9-THC (50 or 100 mg/kg, p.o.)	↓ (Latency to mount) ↓ (No. of mounts) ↓ (Latency to intromit) ↓ (No. of intromissions) ↓ (Latency to ejaculate)	Dalterio *et al.* (1978)
	CBN (50 mg/kg, p.o.)	— (Latency to mount) — (No. of mounts) — (Latency to intromit) — No. of intromissions) — (Latency to ejaculate)	
Mouse	Δ^9-THC (50 mg/kg, p.o.) 2.5 weeks or 7 weeks	↓ (Latency to mount) ↓ (No. of mounts)	Dalterio (1980)

(continued)

TABLE 5.   (*Continued*)

Species	Compound & dose	Sexual behavior	Reference
		↓ (Latency to intromit)	
		↓ (No. of intromissions)	
	CBN (50 mg/kg, p.o.) 2.5 weeks	— (Latency to mount)	
		— (No. of mounts)	
		— (Latency to intromit)	
		— (No. of intromissions)	
Monkey	Δ⁹-THC (2.3–4.8 mg/kg) 3–18 months	— ("Sexual behavior"	Sassenrath & Chapman (1975)

animals (Abel, 1975). Whether these observations of sexual behavior are also part of this difference in consummatory behavior remains to be determined.

EFFECTS ON SPERM AND REPRODUCTIVE ORGANS

Human Studies

Abnormal sperm samples have been reported in several studies. Kolodny and co-workers (1974) reported that 6 out of 17 marihuana smokers they studied had sperm counts below 30 million per ml (no sperm counts were reported for nonmarihuana users). Abnormalities in sperm samples from chronic hashish users were also noted (Issidorides, 1980). Among the reported aberrations were reduced nuclear size, increased condensation of chromatin, disorganization of acrosomal structure, and absence of acrosomes (Hembree *et al.*, 1976; 1980).

Hembree and his co-workers examined sperm production and morphology in 5 chronic marihuana smokers (3 to 5 marihuana cigarettes per week). Subjects entered a hospital setting and during the first 21 days did not smoke marihuana. They were then allowed to smoke increasing amounts of marihuana for the next four weeks with a minimum of 10 cigarettes smoked per day. Four of the 5 subjects had no difficulty sustaining this level and most smoked considerably more (e.g., 31 cigarettes in 1 day). Each cigarette contained 20 mg of Δ^9-THC. This smoking period was followed by a 15-day nonsmoking recovery period.

Sperm concentration or sperm count did not change during the smoking period, but both were significantly lowered (about 58%) during the post-smoking period. Effects on motility were highly variable and did not correlate with sperm count. There was also no significant correlation between decreased sperm production and number of cigarettes smoked. Since these decreases in sperm count were not associated with significant changes in serum testosterone, luteinizing hormone, or follicle-stimulating hormone levels, the authors proposed that the observed decreases in sperm count in the post-smoking period were due to direct suppressant actions of the cannabinoids on the germinal epithelium. These changes during the post-smoking period were accounted for by the time course for human spermatogenesis. Sperm production and transit through the male duct system requires about 87 days. Cannabinoid effects on sperm production occurring during late spermiogenesis would not be observable until 2 weeks after initial cannabinoid use whereas changes would be observed earlier if an effect on release of sperm from manufacturing cells occurred. If interference occurred during initial spermatogonial mitotic divisions, no effect would be observable until a second phase of sperm production occurred, about 3 to 6 months later. The observed alterations during the post-smoking period would thus be consistent with an effect on spermiogenesis, the last phase of sperm production, which occurred in the last 23 days of the cycle, at a time when subjects were smoking marihuana.

The data reported in this study indicate that sperm counts did indeed drop precipitously during the post-smoking period compared to the drug-free period. However, it also appears that sperm count decreased in all subjects during the initial smoking period when less than 10 cigarettes were smoked per session, and increased for 4 of the 5 subjects during the time that unlimited smoking was permitted. These changes were not addressed. Also worth commenting about is the relatively large amount of marihuana consumption involved in this study, the relevance of which to more customary use of marihuana is questionable.

In a subsequent study by Hembree and his associates (1980), another 12 chronic marihuana users were observed. (However, data were reported for 16 subjects. No mention of where these additional 4 subjects were obtained from is indicated in this report.)

As in the previous study, sperm concentration and volume were not altered during the 4-week smoking period, but sperm concentration was significantly lower during the first two weeks after smoking ceased. A return to normal levels occurred by 3-to 4-weeks post-marihuana use. Sperm motility was unaffected for the only subject whose sperm motility was studied. No evidence of abnormal sperm morphology was apparent from either study. The delayed effect on sperm count was attributed to the long period (65 days) normally required for sperm production.

In this study as in the previous one, there were several questionable procedures. In addition, this second study indicated that sexual continence could not be controlled, which may have affected the outcome of both studies.

Studies in Animals

Studies in animals have shown that cannabinoids are distributed to male reproductive organs and there have been several reports of regression of male reproductive organs in animals which appears to be reversible after drug treatment. Studies of changes in male reproductive organs following treatment with cannabinoid compounds are summarized in Table 6.

TABLE 6. Effects of Cannabinoids on Prostate and Testis Weight

Source	Species	Compound	Prostate	Testis	Remarks
Thompson et al., 1973	Rat	Δ^9-THC (50–500 mg/kg/day) Cannabis extract (150–1500 mg/kg/kday) for 119 days, p.o.	↓	↓	Absolute testis weight decreased but testis weight relative to body weight increased. Degeneration in seminiferous tubules. Leydig cells not affected.
Ling et al., 1973		Δ^9-THC (4.16 mg/kg/day) for 5 days, i.p.	—	—	
Thompson et al., 1973	Rhesus monkey	Δ^9-THC (0–500 mg/kg/day) for 28 days, p.o.	—		
		Δ^9-THC (0–45 mg/kg/day) for 28 days, i.v.			
Rosenkrantz, Heyman, & Braude, 1974	Rat	Marihuana smoke (inhalation), acute, 5, and 23 days	—	↑	
Rosenkrantz et al., 1975	Rat	Δ^9-THC (2–50 mg/kg/day) for 28–180 days, p.o.	↓	↑	Absolute prostate weight decreased after 28 and 90 days, but increased

(continued)

TABLE 6. (*Continued*)

Source	Species	Compound	Prostate	Testis	Remarks
Dixit & Lohiya, 1975	Mouse	Cannabis extract (60 mg), i.p.	↓		after 180 days treatment. No evidence of tissue damage.
Vyas & Singh, 1976	Pigeon	Cannabis powder (0.25, 0.5 mg) for 30–90 days		↓	
Harmon et al., 1976	Rat	Δ^9-THC (8 mg/kg) 5 days per week p.o.	↓		
Collu et al., 1975	Rat	Δ^9-THC (1, 10 mg/kg, 3 times/week for 4 weeks i.p.	↓	—	Animals treated beginning at 21 days of age. Prostate weight lower at 10 mg/kg dose. Several vessicle weights not affected.

Reference	Species	Treatment			Remarks
Collu et al., 1975	Rat	Δ⁹-THC (20, 50 μg/day) for 7 days intraventricular	→	—	—	Prostate weights lowered after 20 μg but not after 50 μg.
Okey & Truant, 1975	Rat	Cannabis resin	—	—	
Rosenkrantz & Hayden, 1979	Rat	Marihuana smoke Mexican marihuana Turkish marihuana Placebo impregnated with CBD and CBCH (5 days/week, 17–25 days)	→	→↑	Absolute testis weights decreased, relative testis weights increased, for Turkish marihuana, seminiferous tubule degeneration.
				→	Absolute testis weights decreased but relative weights not affected with CBD.
Purohit et al., 1979	Rat	Δ⁹-THC 10 mg/kg/day CBN 10 mg/kg/day for 10 days, s.c.	→ →		

As indicated by the table, there is reasonably good consensus that cannabinoids reduce prostate weights. The effect on testis weight is inconsistent, with effects ranging from increased, to no changes, to decreased weight.

Despite the inconsistency of reports concerning cannabinoid-induced changes in testis weight, consistent changes in testis function have been observed in animals following treatment with cannabinoids, even in the absence of weight changes.

Daily administration of cannabis extract (12.5 mg/kg, s.c.) for 30 days caused seminiferous tubule degeneration and degeneration of spermatogonia, spermatocytes, spermatids, and spermatozoa in dogs (Dixit, 1975).

Vyas and Singh (1976) observed seminiferous tubule degeneration and marked reductions in spermatogonia and spermatocyte levels in pigeons after cannabinoid exposure. By 60 days of daily administration of 0.25 mg/kg, aspermia was evident. Absence of sperm was also produced after only 30 days of daily treatment with 0.5 mg/kg. Degenerative changes in spermatogonia (chromatolysis, cytolysis) and spermatocytes were also evident.

Rosenkrantz and Hayden (1979) observed seminiferous tubule degeneration in rats exposed to Turkish marihuana smoke and placebo smoke containing CBD or CBCH, but not in animals exposed to an amount of Δ^9-THC three times greater than CBD or CBCH. Degenerative changes in spermatocytes and spermatids were also visible following exposure to Turkish marihuana smoke.

Rosenkrantz and co-workers have also reported that seminiferous tubule degeneration occurred after treatment with doses of 50 to 500 mg/kg/day Δ^9-THC but not with doses of 2 to 50 mg/kg/day (Thompson *et al.*, 1973; Rosenkrantz *et al.*, 1975).

Zimmerman and Zimmerman (1979) injected (i.p.) mice with 5 or 10 mg/kg/day of Δ^9-THC for five days. Drug treatment resulted in a dose-related increase in abnormal sperm (e.g., heads lacking hooks, banana-shaped heads, amorphous heads, folded heads). Mice treated with 10 or 25 mg/kg CBN daily also had dose-related increases in abnormal sperm morphology. Comparable treatment with CBD did not result in such changes. A subsequent cytogenic examination (Zimmerman *et al.*, 1980) noted a 3- to 5-fold increase in chromosomal translocations. However, the significance of these observations is dubious as a result of the high mortality rate (>50%) in animals receiving these relatively low doses. Changes in sperm morphology, for instance, may have been due to secondary effects of drug administration.

In yet another study (Huang *et al.*, 1980), rats exposed to marihuana smoke (30 exposures in 30 days to 4 puffs daily, or 75 exposures in 90 days to 16 puffs daily) had fewer epididymal sperm compared to controls. Although regarded as "significant," the statistical significance level was >.5 <.10, a level dismissed as nonsignificant by these same authors in discussing the decreased body weights of these animals. The importance of monitoring body weight, however, is not without merit since many of the effects on reproductive organs noted in other studies may be a secondary function of marihuana-related decreases in food consumption and consequent undernutrition.

In this regard, the brief report by Harmon and co-workers (1976) is worth noting. In this study, rats were treated with Δ^9-THC (8 mg/kg/5 days per week) for 5 weeks. A control group received the vehicle only, and in addition was pair-fed to the drug-treated group, such that these animals were allotted food equal to that consumed by the drug-treated group. When drug-treated animals were compared to this control group, spermatogenesis was affected in only two animals relative to controls.

In vitro studies have shown that cannabinoids can inhibit protein and nucleic acid synthesis and glucose metabolism in the rat testis. Inhibition is greatest in seminiferous tubule cells (Jakubovic *et al.*, 1979). Since protein and nucleic acid synthesis and metabolism of glucose are involved in spermatogenesis, inhibition of these processes could account for the decreased sperm production associated with cannabinoid exposure in animals.

In summary, studies in which cannabinoids have been administered to animals are quite consistent in demonstrating adverse effects on sperm production. These effects are similar to those reported in humans. On the other hand, these studies in both humans and animals are poorly controlled and are subject to alternative explanations, the most simple of which is that these effects are in large part due to drug-related undernutrition. In only one instance was an adequate control procedure instituted for this possibility and when this was done, the result was not convincing as far as adverse effects on sperm production are concerned.

In addition, the potential significance of the reported effects on sperm production is unclear since there is no indication that dominant lethal mutation rates are increased as a result of chronic treatment with cannabinoids. Legator and his co-workers (1976), for example, did not observe any affects on fertility, number of implantations per female, number of corpor lutea, preimplantation losses, or resorption rates following administration of Δ^9-THC for 4 weeks prior to and during mating. Although one or more of these parameters might have been affected if drug treatment were longer, there is no evidence from either the clinical or the preclinical literature to support this possibility.

Effects on Hormones

Testosterone

Testosterone, the male sex hormone, is primarily produced (95%) by the Leydig cells located in the testis. The adrenals produce the remaining amount of testosterone. About 7 mg of testosterone is produced by the adult male per day (Rose, 1975).

Testosterone levels in the adult male range between 400 and 1200 ng%, although levels as low as 275 and as high as 1500 ng% have been noted. Nearly all (96–98%) of the testosterone in the blood is bound to sex steroid binding globulin, leaving only 2 to 4% free to interact with target tissues (Rose, 1975).

Testosterone production is controlled by luteinizing hormone (LH), which is also known as interstitial cell stimulating hormone (ICSH), secreted by the pituitary. However, luteinizing hormone levels do not exhibit the same diurnal cycle as testosterone levels, and some drugs that affect testosterone levels do not appear to affect luteinizing hormone levels. On the other hand, there does seem to be a general negative feedback relationship between luteinizing hormone levels and testosterone production.

Plasma testosterone levels exhibit a marked diurnal cycle with about a 40% difference between the high and low levels (Rose, 1975). Even when samples are taken at the same time of day, variability in some men may reach 20–25%. The diurnal cycle and large variability between and within subjects underscores the importance of longitudinal measurements conducted at the same time of day in the same individuals. The most appropriate design for such studies is of necessity a "within subjects" protocol wherein each individual serves as his own control.

Currently, there is no consensus regarding the effects of marihuana on testosterone production (see Table 7).

Decreased plasma testosterone levels were reported by Kolodny and co-workers (1974) in men who had been smoking marihuana at least 4 times a week for 6 months. Comparisons were made with 20 nonusers matched for age and cigarette use. Plasma testosterone samples were collected in the early morning on different days, at least 1 month apart. When marihuana users were given human chorionic gonadotropin, which stimulates testosterone production, testosterone levels increased by over 120%, indicating functional Leydig cell capacity. Following a two-week period of marihuana abstinence, testosterone levels also increased. Sexual functioning was reported as not being affected in any subjects except for one.

In contrast to this report, most other studies have not found any evidence that marihuana use affects testosterone levels. Mendelson and co-workers (1978), for example, divided 27 marihuana users into "casual" (mean prior usage of 5 years, 11 times per month) and "heavy" (mean usage for 5 years, 42 marihuana cigarettes per month) categories. During the first 5 days of the study, baseline measures of testosterone were obtained. During the next 21 days, subjects smoked marihuana. During a final 5-day period, no marihuana was smoked. Plasma samples were obtained once

TABLE 7. Levels of Testosterone Associated with Use of Marihuana

Source	Users	Nonusers	Comments
Kolodny et al., 1974	416 ng%	742 ng%	Subjects (N = 20) smoked average of 9 marihuana cigarettes per week. Controls (N = 20) were non-marihuana users.
Cushman, 1975	639 ng%	633 ng%	Marihuana users (N = 25) smoked average of 5 marihuana cigarettes per week. Controls (N = 13) were nonmarihuana users.
Mendelson et al., 1974	Before usage Casual (988 ng%) Heavy (1115 ng%)	After usage 800–1000 ng%[a] 1000–1110 ng%[a]	No significant changes in testosterone levels after 21 days of smoking marihuana.
Schaefer et al., 1975	867 ng%	793 ng%	Subjects (N = 12) tested 90 min after smoking cigarettes containing Δ^9THC (20 mg).
Kolodny et al., 1976	754 ng%	533 ng%	Subjects (N = 20) tested 3 hrs after smoking 1 marihuana cigarette.
Mendelson et al., 1978	970%	994%	Baseline testosterone range (112–2319 ng%) rose after smoking marihuana for 26 days (267–2235).

[a]Data estimated from figures.

per day in the early morning. No significant changes in testosterone levels were found for either the casual or the heavy marihuana users during the study nor did testosterone levels differ between the two groups.

Testosterone levels were not significantly affected in a study reported by Schaefer and his associates (1975). In this report, 12 men, described as "varying from occasional to habitual users of marihuana," lived on a research ward for 5 days. On the first day, baseline testosterone data were collected. On the next three days, placebo, 10 mg, and 20 mg of Δ^9-THC were administered in marihuana cigarettes. On the fifth day, 20 mg Δ^9-THC was again administered, and blood samples were obtained 30 minutes before and 90 minutes after smoking. (Since the average marihuana cigarette contained about 5 mg Δ^9-THC at the time of this study, subjects smoked the equivalent of about 4 marihuana cigarettes during this final phase). When concentrations of testosterone before and after the 20 mg dose were compared, there was a small, but statistically significant reduction (8.5%) in testosterone levels which the authors suggest may have been due to the normal circadian rhythm for this hormone. The authors also point out that the plasma testosterone levels in their subjects ranged from 445 to 1213 ng% even though some of these subjects were considered "heavy" marihuana users and that these levels fell well within the range considered "normal" for adult men.

Cushman (1975) compared plasma testosterone levels in 25 marihuana smokers (average time of usage was 2.8 years, average amount of use was 5 marihuana cigarettes weekly) with 13 non-marihuana users. Using the same "between subjects" design as Kolodny and co-workers (1974), Cushman (1975) did not observe any significant differences in testosterone levels between the two groups. Average testosterone level for the marihuana users was 639 ng%, which is within the range of normal testosterone values.

A failure to detect marihuana-induced changes in testosterone levels has also been reported by Hembree and his co-workers (1976).

Since the Kolodny study (1974) is the only one to report marihuana-related changes in plasma testosterone, a few comments regarding the procedures used in that study are warranted. These comments also have a bearing on the research conducted in connection with other substances as well as on research discussed in subsequent sections.

One major criticism directed at the Kolodny study was the

manner in which blood sampling was performed. Since two samples, drawn one month apart, are generally insufficient to produce reliable data, Kolodny's report of marihuana-related decreases in plasma testosterone could have been due to sampling error. The possibility of sampling error is also suggested by the fact that the levels of testosterone reported in this study (416 ng%) were somewhat lower than those reported in other studies, but were still within the range considered "normal."

A second criticism is the use of a "between subjects" design for studying marihuana effects on testosterone levels. Such a design is likely to be less sensitive than the "within subjects" design used by Mendelson *et al.* (1978) and Schaefer *et al.* (1975). The considerable variability both between and within subjects underscores the importance of repeated longitudinal measures conducted at the same time of day in the same subjects for accurate assessment of changes in testosterone levels.

In answer to the criticisms concerning type of design and sampling method, Kolodny (1976) conducted a second study using a "within subjects" protocol and a procedure in which subjects were sampled at 15, 30, 60, 120, and 180 minutes after marihuana smoking. As in their previous study, testosterone levels were significantly reduced after smoking (at 30, 120, and 180 minutes) compared to a control nonsmoking period.

To examine this effect on hourly plasma testosterone levels, Mendelson and co-workers (1974) conducted a comparable study in which 13 men who reported smoking for 5 to 9 years (20 to 60 cigarettes/month) were evaluated using the same three-phase design as used in their previous study. Blood samples were obtained on an hourly basis on the last day of the baseline phase, the twenty-first day of marihuana smoking, and on the third day after marihuana cessation. Contrary to Kolodny's (1976) results, plasma testosterone levels were not affected even when measured on an hourly basis.

In summary, there is no consistency in the data regarding marihuana's effects on testosterone levels in adult males. Although the results of one of the studies reporting decreases in testosterone related to marihuana use can be faulted on methodological grounds, the other study is less subject to criticism, and it is difficult to resolve the discrepancy between it and other studies in the area.

Studies in Animals

In contrast to studies in humans, studies in rats have reported consistent cannabinoid-induced decreases in plasma testosterone levels. These studies are summarized in Table 8.

Although impairment of Leydig cell function could account for these results, the data examining this possibility are inconsistent. For example, Dixit and co-workers (1974) observed regression of Leydig cells in mice following chronic exposure to cannabis extract. Vyas and Singh (1976), on the other hand, did not observe any changes in Leydig cells in pigeons following chronic treatment with cannabis despite extensive damage to other testicular tissue.

Basal Leydig cell production of testosterone was not affected by Δ^9-THC, CBN, CBD, or CBG *in vitro* (Jakubovic *et al.*, 1979; Dalterio *et al.*, 1977). Decreased testosterone production *in vitro* by testicular microsomes obtained from rats treated acutely with Δ^9-THC (2 or 10 mg/kg) has been reported, however, by List and his co-workers (List, 1977). List also observed increased liver metabolism of testosterone which could account, in part, for cannabinoid-related decreases in circulating testosterone levels in animals.

Functional Leydig cell capacity is also suggested by several studies in both humans (Kolodny, 1974) and animals (Purohit, 1979) which reported increased testosterone levels following administration of human chorionic gonadotropin to marihuana users or animals treated with cannabinoids. Dalterio and her co-workers (1977), on the other hand, reported an inhibition of testosterone production by testes when incubated with Δ^9-THC and human chorionic gonadotropin. The explanation for these discrepancies has yet to be accounted for.

Luteinizing Hormone

Although there are some inconsistencies in the negative feedback model proposed to exist between pituitary release of luteiniz-

Table 8. Effects of Cannabinoids on Plasma Testosterone and Luteinizing Hormone Levels in Animals

Source	Species	Compound	Testosterone	LH	Remarks
Symons et al., 1976	Rat	Δ⁹-THC (5 mg/kg/twice weekly) for 6 weeks, i.m.	↓	↓	Δ⁹-THC decreased pituitary responsiveness to LH–RH
		Δ⁹-THC (5 mg/kg) acute, i.m.	↓	↓	
Maskarinec et al., 1978	Rat	Cannabis extract	↓		Testosterone not lowered by Δ⁹-THC except at 50 mg/kg dose, cannabis extract containing 5 mg/kg Δ⁹-THC decreased testosterone by same amount
		Δ⁹-THC (1–50 mg/kg)	↓		
Collu et al., 1975	Rat	Δ⁹-THC (1, 10 mg/kg) 3 times per week for 1 month, i.p.		↓ ↓	

Reference	Species	Treatment		
Collu, 1976	Rat	Δ⁹-THC (20, 50 μg/day) for 7 days, intraventricular		← —
Harmon et al., 1976	Rat	Δ⁹-THC (8 mg/kg) 5 days/week	→	
Purohit et al., 1979	Rat	Δ⁹-THC (10 mg/kg/day), CBN (10 mg/kg/day) for 10 days, s.c.	→	
Dalterio et al., 1978	Mouse	Δ⁹-THC (50 or 100 mg/kg acute, p.o.)	→	→ —
		CBN (50 mg/kg, acute, p.o.)	—	—
Dalterio 1980	Mouse	Δ⁹-THC (50 mg/kg, 3 weeks, 3 times per week, p.o.)	—	—
		Δ⁹-THC (50 mg/kg, 7 weeks, 3 times per week, p.o.)	—	—

ing hormone (LH) and Leydig cell production of testosterone, stimulation of testosterone is generally presumed to be governed by luteinizing hormone.

Human Studies

Kolodny and his co-workers (1974) reported that luteinizing hormone levels did not differ significantly in marihuana users compared to nonmarihuana users. However, in a second study by this group, luteinizing hormone levels were decreased 180 minutes after smoking marihuana.

In contrast to this result, significant changes in luteinizing hormone levels in adult men have not been found in other studies comparing marihuana and nonmarihuana users, or in longitudinal studies of changes in this hormone following marihuana usage (Mendelson *et al.*, 1978; 1974).

The decrease in luteinizing hormone levels at 180 minutes after smoking marihuana as reported by Kolodny (1974) is difficult to account for, since a decrease in testosterone levels was also noted in these same subjects at this time (see above). A decrease in one of these hormones should have been accompanied by an increase in the other as a consequence of the negative feedback relationship between the two. Since these data are contradicted by other studies and are contrary to what might be expected on the basis of the relation between luteinizing hormone and testosterone production, the most likely explanation for this finding at this time is sampling error.

Animal Studies

Effects of cannabinoids on luteinizing hormone levels in male animals have not been consistent (see Table 8). Symons and his co-workers (1976) and Dalterio and her co-workers both reported a decrease in luteinizing hormone levels associated with a decrease in testosterone levels (Dalterio, 1980).

Biological Significance of Observations

In general there is little indication that marihuana usage in humans or animals adversely affects male reproductive function in any biologically meaningful way. Anecdotal information suggests that marihuana increases sexual enjoyment or performance but there is no unequivocal evidence to support this belief. Studies of male sexual behavior in animals are compromised because of the well-known effect of the cannabinoids to suppress motor activity and consummatory behavior in general. Methodological problems inherent in many of the studies conducted in animals to date (e.g., testing males with a female that is not in estrus) make conclusions regarding decreased sexual performance equivocal at best.

The reported abnormalities in sperm samples in human marihuana users are consistent, but methodological problems also compromise these observations. Although many studies were conducted in research wards, there is no indication that these subjects were permitted or not permitted to receive female visitors with whom they may have engaged in sex, or whether in fact they masturbated during the study period. In such cases, semen volume and concentration may have been affected. Whereas abnormal sperm would not result from such confounding factors, reports of such abnormalities in marihuana smokers have not been consistent.

Studies in animals are not consistent in demonstrating adverse effects on male sex organs. More important, in virtually every study there is a basic confounding between drug administration and food deprivation. Since cannabinoid compounds reliably produce weight losses in animals by decreasing food and water consumption, the possible role of undernutrition as contributing to the reported effects should be considered. Although testes weight does not always decrease following food deprivation, in some instances testes may become severely atrophic following food restriction (Mulinas, 1941). The variability in such observations is similar to the variability seen in connection with marihuana's effects on male sex organs.

The reported effects on sperm volume and morphology are also subject to debate since there is no evidence to date that off-spring sired by male marihuana users are affected in any way.

The reported effects of marihuana use on testosterone levels and luteinizing hormone levels are inconsistent. Even when "statistically significant" decreases have been reported, the "biological significance" of such decreases are moot since levels are invariably within ranges considered normal for adult males. Moreover, the role of testosterone in male sexual behavior is still problematical. For example, testosterone does not restore sexual performance in castrated animals much beyond precastration levels (Davidson, 1972). Castration also does not immediately result in absence of mating behavior. In some instances, men who were legally castrated continued to engage in sexual intercourse for many years after castration. On the other hand, testosterone is, of course, essential for maintenance of male sex organs and secondary sex characteristics but levels of this hormone must be considerably lower than what has been observed thus far in human and in most animal studies, for libido to be affected significantly.

FEMALE REPRODUCTION

During the 19th century cannabis was frequently recommended by physicians in the treatment of menstrual disorders such as menorrhagia and dysmenorrhea. Brown (1883) commented that in his clinical experience cannabis rarely failed to relieve menorrhagia and he considered the drug as a "specific" for the condition.

Cannabis has also been used for centuries as a folk remedy to facilitate childbirth. Early medical trials in England, shortly after introduction of the drug to that country, indicated that it increased the force of uterine contractions and shortened labor considerably (Grigor, 1852).

Despite these and related endorsements and cannabis' long standing use in childbirth, clinicians were generally reluctant to use the drug in their practices because of difficulties in controlling dosage and other related problems (Abel, 1980b).

Although there have been many recent studies of the effects of cannabinoids in humans and animals, very little attention has been devoted to an examination of the drug's effects on female reproductive function. Current studies of marihuana's effects in women, for example, are nonexistent. What little information is available is derived primarily from studies in animals.

Human Studies

The only study concerning marihuana's effects on reproductive function in women was reported by Kolodny and his co-workers (1979). Marihuana users had shorter menstrual cycles (26.8 days) compared to nonmarihuana users (28.8 days), and had more menstrual cycles that were either anovulatory or characterized by a shorter luteal phase (38.3% *vs.* 12.5%). Hormonal profiles did not differentiate marihuana users from nonusers in terms of serum luteinizing hormone, follicle stimulating hormone, estrogen, or progesterone levels. However, serum prolactin levels were significantly lower and serum testosterone levels were significantly higher in marihuana users.

These results, as acknowledged by the authors themselves, should only be considered preliminary. Among the confounding variables noted by the authors is the more than twofold greater alcohol consumption by marihuana users. Since alcohol use is also associated with menstrual irregularities (Abel, 1980b), differences between the marihuana users and nonusers could have been due to this variable. Another variable on which these women differed was sexual activity, with marihuana users being more sexually active than nonusers. The significance of this variable with respect to the observed differences, however, is unknown. Finally, both the validity of combining luteal-phase inadequacy and anovulatory cycles, and the relevance of either measure to fertility, are also questionable.

Studies in Animals

The effects of cannabinoids on female reproductive organs and function has been examined in a number of studies. As in the case of reproductive studies in males, many of these studies are poorly designed and are confounded by lack of attention to possible side effects of cannabinoid administration on food and water consumption.

Sexual Behavior

Facilitation of lordosis in estrogen-primed females by acute administration of Δ^9-THC has been reported in two studies (Gordon *et al.*, 1978; Turley *et al.*, 1981). Chronic treatment did not affect the lordosis response. This result was not affected by concurrent antiestrogen treatment and differed from the effects of progesterone. The authors concluded that the most likely explanation for this result was a direct, nonhormonal effect of the drug on the central nervous system mechanisms underlying this behavior. This is an interesting observation which warrants further study. It would be important, for instance, to determine if this effect was due to enhancement of motor response underlying lordosis, or to some effect on motivational mechanisms underlying sexual activity. In any case, these two reports are unusual in that they offer evidence for the enhancement of sexual activity in conjunction with marihuana usage.

Ovulation

Several studies have consistently shown that cannabinoids adversely affect ovulation in animals. A dose-related inhibition of ovulation in rabbits was observed following administration of Δ^9-THC (0.3 to 5 mg/kg, i.m.) (Asch *et al.*, 1979). Animals treated with 2.5 or 5 mg/kg doses failed to ovulate at all. However, ovulation was not inhibited when human chorionic gonadotropin was administered along with Δ^9-THC. Ovulation was eliminated in rats and mice after daily administration of cannabis extract. By day 64 of treatment, ovaries were reduced in size and there was a diminution of ova (Asch, 1979).

Daily administration of Δ^9-THC (1 to 2.5 mg/kg) did not affect ovulation in monkeys during the time of drug treatment but all animals had anovulatory cycles (confirmed by laparascopy) in the cycle following drug treatment (Sassenrath & Chapman, 1975; Smith *et al.*, 1980). These anovulatory cycles were associated with below normal luteinizing and follicle stimulating hormone levels.

EFFECTS ON HORMONES

Luteinizing and Follicle Stimulating Hormone

Δ^9-THC has consistently been shown to depress plasma luteinizing hormone levels in female animals (see Table 9).

This decrease occurs in both ovariectomized (Besch *et al.*, 1977; Marks, 1973; Smith *et al.*, 1979; Tyrey, 1978) and intact animals (Nir *et al.*, 1973; Ayalon *et al.*, 1977; Chakravarty *et al.*, 1975). Duration of effect is related to dosage, and is likely a main reason anovulation occurs following treatment with cannabinoids.

A single administration of Δ^9-THC (10 mg/kg, i.p.), on the day of proestrus, suppressed ovulation in rats by inhibiting the usual luteinizing hormone surge initiating ovulation (Nir *et al.*, 1973; Ayalon *et al.*, 1977; Burstein and Raz, 1972). Inhibition of episodic luteinizing hormone release in ovariectomized rats by Δ^9-THC has also been reported (Smith *et al.*, 1980).

Administration of luteinizing hormone-releasing hormone increases luteinizing hormone levels in ovariectomized animals treated with Δ^9-THC and restores ovulation in animals made anovulatory by Δ^9-THC (Asch *et al.*, 1979; Ayalon *et al.*, 1977). Pituitary responsiveness of luteinizing hormone-releasing hormone thus does not appear to be affected by the drug.

Instead of acting at the pituitary, Δ^9-THC appears to affect hypothalamic mechanisms which release luteinizing hormone-

TABLE 9. Effects of Cannabinoids on Blood LH Levels in Females

Source	Species	Compound	Effects on LH	Comments
Asch et al., 1979	Rabbit	Δ⁹-THC (0.3–5 mg/kg, i.m.)	↓	
Besch et al., 1977	Rhesus monkey	Δ⁹-THC (0.6–5 mg/kg, i.m.)	↓	Decrease not dose-related but duration of effect was dose-related
Chakravarty et al., 1979	Rat	Δ⁹-THC (5–10 mg/kg, i.p. for 10 days)	↓	Pituitary levels of LH were higher than in controls
Kolodny et al., 1979	Women	Marihuana 4 days per week for at least 6 months	—	Comparison of marihuana and non-marihuana users
Marks, 1973	Rat	Δ⁹-THC (10 mg/kg, i.p.)	↓	Dose-dependent decreases
Nir et al., 1973	Rat	Δ⁹-THC (10 mg/kg, i.p.)	↓	
Smith et al., 1979	Rhesus monkey	Δ⁹-THC (0.3–5 mg/kg, i.m.)	↓	Dose-dependent decreases in LH, duration of effect also dose-related
Tyrey, 1978	Rat	Δ⁹-THC (0.5–8.0 mg/kg, i.v)	↓	Duration was dose-dependent

releasing hormone. This likelihood is supported by the dose-dependent decrease in hypothalamic content of this releasing hormone following chronic administration of Δ^9-THC (Chakravarty, 1979).

Another possible mechanism by which cannabinoids affect luteinizing hormone is by affecting prostaglandins. Prostaglandins are able to stimulate release of luteinizing hormone, and inhibition of prostaglandin synthesis results in suppression of luteinizing hormone. The site of action for these effects of prostaglandin is believed to be in the hypothalamus, and prostaglandin is believed to be involved in the release of luteinizing hormone-releasing hormone from the hypothalamus.

Support for this hypothesis is derived from studies showing that Δ^9-THC inhibits prostagandin synthesis *in vitro* (Burstein and Raz, 1972). However, Ayalon *et al.* (1977) did not observe any changes in hypothalamic prostaglandin content in proestrus rats following administration of Δ^9-THC. In addition, Δ^9-THC was unable to affect prostaglandin-induced increases in luteinizing hormone.

Cannabinoids may also affect ovulation by decreasing the sensitivity of the ovary to luteinizing hormone. Δ^9-THC and Nembutal both block ovulation and reduce ovarian prostaglandin content. Administration of luteinizing hormone at doses (2.5 μg) that are able to overcome the Nembutal block and restore prostaglandin content are only partially capable of overcoming the Δ^9-THC-induced inhibition of ovulation and depression of prostaglandins. Higher doses of luteinizing hormone (10 μg), on the other hand, were able to reverse the ovulation block and depression of prostaglandin (Ayalon *et al.*, 1977).

Effects on follicle-stimulating hormone following administration of cannabinoids have not been studied to the same extent as effects on luteinizing hormone. Relevant studies are indicated in Table 10.

Although there is a tendency for these hormone levels to be depressed following exposure to Δ^9-THC, there are too few studies from which to derive any generalizations.

TABLE 10.   Effects of Cannabinoids on Blood FSH Levels in Females

Source	Species	Compound	Effects of FSH levels	Comments
Smith *et al.*, 1979	Rhesus monkey	Δ^9-THC, (0.3–5 mg/kg, i.m.)	↓	Decreases occurred only with 2.5 and 5.0 mg/kg doses
Kolodny *et al.*, 1979	Women	Marihuana 4 days per week for 6 months	—	Comparison of marihuana and non-marihuana users
Chakravarty *et al.*, 1979	Rat	Δ^9-THC (5–10 mg/kg, i.p., for 10 days)	↓	Higher pituitary FSH levels in drug-treated animals

Estrogen

The report of gynecomastia in three young adult marihuana users touched off speculation that marihuana might have estrogenic properties. In describing these three cases, for example, Harmon and Alipoulios (1972) commented on the similarities between Δ^9-THC and estradiol, and hypothesized that marihuana might act directly on the breast or might exert its effect through prolactin.

Other studies, however, have not corroborated the original report or found any reliable indication that cannabinoids do possess estrogenic properties.

For example, a study of gynecomastia patients among a population of U.S. soldiers stationed in Germany did not find any significant relationship between gynecomastia and marihuana use (Cates and Pope, 1977). In another instance, observation of gynecomastia in a marihuana user could not be attributed to marihuana use since the condition had existed since adolescence, several years prior to marihuana usage (Kolodny *et al.*, 1974).

The total absence of corroborating reports of gynecomastia in marihuana smokers thus suggests that the observation of gynecomastia in marihuana smokers originally reported by Harmon and Alipoulios was merely coincidental. Nevertheless, there have been numerous studies investigating the possibility of estrogen-like properties for cannabinoid compounds.

These studies have adopted one of two strategies in examining this issue. One strategy has involved bioassay tests in whole animals to determine if cannabinoids promote growth of estrogen-responsive tissues such as the uterus. The second strategy has involved *in vitro* binding tests to determine if cannabinoids compete with estrogens for specific receptor sites.

Studies of changes in uterus and ovarian weights in animals following chronic exposure to cannabinoids do not support the hypothesis that these compounds possess estrogenic properties. These studies are summarized in Table 11.

Ovarian weight is generally decreased following chronic can-

TABLE 11. Effects of Cannabinoids on Estrogen Sensitive Organs

Source	Species	Treatment	Uterus wt.	Ovarian wt.	Remarks
Dixit et al., 1975	Rat	Cannabis extract (25 mg/kg/day)	↓	↓	Cellular irregularities in ovaries, uterus and vaginal tissue
	Mice	Cannabis extract (40 mg/kg/day) for 64 days (i.p.)	↓	↓	
Fujimoto et al., 1979	Rat	Δ^9-THC (1–25 mg/kg/day) Cannabis extract (3–75 mg/kg/day) for 72 days (p.o.)	↓	↓	Dose-related decreases in both absolute and relative uterus and ovarian weights. Atrophic and endometrial glands. Uterine and ovarian weights returned to normal by 30 days after drug treatment
Okey & Truant, 1975	Rat	Cannabis resin diet		↓	
Rosenkrantz et al., 1974	Rat	Marihuana cigarette smoke, acute, 5, 23 days	—	—	
Rosenkrantz et al., 1975	Rat	Δ^9-THC (2, 10, 50 mg/kg/day) for 28, 90, 180 days (p.o.)			

Reference	Species	Treatment	Effect	Comments
Solomon et al., 1976	Rat	Δ⁹-THC (1–10 mg/kg/day) 14 days (i.p.)	↑	Increases in uterine weight were dose-related. Histological examination (Solomon et al., 1977) revealed Δ⁹-THC-induced growth of uterine surface epithelium, endometrial glands, and stroma and the myometrium
Rosenkrantz & Hayden, 1979	Rat	Turkish marihuana smoke / Placebo smoke containing CBD	↑ / ↓	Not dose-related
Thompson et al., 1973	Rat	Δ⁹-THC (50–500 mg/kg/day) / Cannabis extract (150–1500 mg/kg/day for 119 days (p.o.)	↓ / → →	
Thompson et al., 1974	Rhesus monkey	Δ⁹-THC (0–500 mg/kg/day) for 28 days (p.o.)	—	
Virgo, 1979	Rat	Δ⁹-THC	↑	Data reanalyzed by Solomon & Schoenfeld, 1980

nabinoid exposure. Fujimoto and co-workers (1979) reported that
Δ^9-THC produced dose-dependent decreases in both absolute and
relative ovarian weights. Weights returned to normal by 30 days
after drug exposure.

Cannabinoid effects on uterus weights are less consistent (see
Table 11). Some studies have reported increased weights following
cannabinoid exposure, whereas decreases and no changes have
been noted in other studies.

Cannabinoids cause relaxation of uterine tissues (Bose *et al.*,
1963) and have a dehydrating effect on the prepubertal rat uterus
(Chakravarty *et al.*, 1975), but do not affect estradiol binding in
mammary or uterine tissues from rats (Okey & Truant, 1975; Okey &
Bondy, 1977, 1978). There is also no significant competition between
Δ^9-THC and estradiol in uterine tissue taken from women who have
had hysterectomies (Gordon *et al.*, 1978), or in nonhuman primate
uterus. In one of the instances in which competition was reported
(Rawitch *et al.*, 1977), the procedures were criticized, e.g., "specific
activity of the ^{14}C-Δ^9-THC (was) so low that its binding to estrogen
receptors . . . could not possibly be determined" (Fujimoto *et al.*,
1979). The second study (Shoemaker & Harmon, 1977) was presented as a brief abstract and not enough information was available to
assess procedures adequately.

In summary, cannabinoid compounds do not appear to possess
estrogenic activity.

Progesterone

Cannabinoids produce a number of effects on ovarian progesterone, but there is no clear pattern discernible. Relatively high
amounts of Δ^9-THC accumulate in the corpora lutea (Freudenthal *et
al.*, 1972), but there is no competition between Δ^9-THC and progesterone receptors in the ovary (Smith *et al.*, 1979). Corpora luteal
cell diameters decreased, and vacuolated luteal cell numbers increased, following chronic exposure of mice to cannabis extract
(Cates & Pope, 1977). Rat luteal cell progesterone synthesis was also
inhibited by marihuana *in vitro* (Burstein *et al.*, 1979). A decrease in

luteal phase progesterone levels was similarly noted in female marihuana users.

In contrast to these observations, no changes in progesterone synthesis were reported in two studies: Plasma progesterone levels and luteal-phase lengths were not affected in nonhuman primates following daily administration of Δ^9-THC (2.5 mg/kg/day, i.m.) (Asch *et al.*, 1979), and in rabbits, plasma progesterone levels were not affected following injection with Δ^9-THC during the luteal phase in conjunction with human chorionogonadotropin challenge (Asch *et al.*, 1979).

Prolactin

In males, cannabinoids have been reported to produce both dose-related increases (Collu, *et al.*, 1975; Daley *et al.*, 1974) and decreases (Kramer & Ben-David, 1974) in prolactin in rats. Results in female animals have been more consistent. Serum prolactin levels in adult female rats were considerably lower following an injection (i.p.) of Δ^9-THC (50 mg/kg) on day of estrus (23 *vs.* 172 ng/ml) (Chakravarty *et al.*, 1975). Prolactin levels were also reduced when Δ^9-THC was administered on day of proestrus (Ayalon *et al.*, 1977). Bromley and co-workers (1978) reported that whereas sucking caused a rapid rise in serum prolactin in rats, administration of Δ^9-THC (1.25 or 4 mg/kg) caused a considerable depression of the sucking-induced increase in serum prolactin. In this study, blood samples were removed via an indwelling catheter and were monitored at 30, 60, and 120 minutes after drug administration. These and other related studies are summarized in Table 12.

This effect on prolactin may account for the inhibition of milk production in lactating animals. Rat pups raised by mothers treated with cannabinoids during pregnancy have a higher postnatal mortality rate than other pups. Examination of their stomachs indicated that these pups were not receiving milk. Cross-fostering procedures, by which pups born to drug-treated dams were placed with nondrug treated dams, reduced the mortality rate. This effect,

TABLE 12.   Effects of Cannabinoids on Serum Prolactin Levels in Females

Species	Dose and route	Prolactin levels	Reference
Human	Smoking	↓	Kolodny *Et al.*, 1974
Rat	Δ⁹-THC (50 mg/kg, i.p.)	↓	Chakravarty *et al.*, 1975
Rat	Δ⁹-THC (2 mg/rat, i.p.)	↓	Ayalon *et al.*, 1977
Rat	Δ⁹-THC (5–10 mg/kg, i.p.)	↓	Chakravarty *et al.*, 1979
Rat	Δ⁹-THC (1.25, 4.0 mg/g, i.v.)	↓	Bromley *et al.*, 1978
Mouse	Δ⁹-THC (25 mg/kg, s.c.)	↓	Raine *et al.*, 1978

however, appears to be dose-related and is not necessarily due to prolactin inhibition, since it is also possible that milk production could be due to some direct effect on the mammary glands.

SUMMARY AND CONCLUSIONS

Centuries after marihuana's effects on libido and sexual performance were first commented on, there is still little reliable information about how marihuana affects human sexuality. Whereas marihuana usage is undeniably associated with increased sexual activity for many people, this association is more likely the result of a particular life-style of sensation-seeking than one related to the pharmacological effects of the drug. Not unexpectedly, the relation between marihuana use and sex appears to be dose-related. At lower doses, factors of "set" and "setting" are predominant, whereas at higher doses, pharmacological factors assume more importance. Determining threshold levels for these effects in conjunction with sexual behavior is not possible since there are no laboratory studies available from which to make such generalizations. Studies in animals are unlikely to shed much light on marihuana's effects on sexual behavior because marihuana tends to decrease all forms of consummatory behavior in subhumans.

Considerable effort has been expended in attempting to characterize marihuana's effects on hormones involved in reproduction. Although initial studies suggested that marihuana lowered testosterone levels in men, these studies were not corroborated and at present the weight of the evidence suggests that there is no biologically or statistically significant change in testosterone levels in men following marihuana usage. Although the weight of the evidence does indicate that sperm production is adversely affected by marihuana usage in men, the biological significance of this observation is unclear since there is no evidence for marihuana-related dominant lethal mutations or any other effects on male reproductive function associated with its usage.

Studies in animals can be cited to support or refute marihuana's effects on reproductive function since much of these data are inconsistent. Perhaps one reason for this inconsistency is the absence of important control procedures to evaluate drug effects. For example, one of the important effects of cannabinoid exposure in animals is decreased consumption of food and water. Reproductive function is definitely related to nutritional status, and if adverse effects on male reproductive organs or function occur in conjunction with administration of cannabinoids, it is important to determine if these effects are due to the pharmacological actions of cannabinoids on reproductive function or to secondary effects such as undernutrition.

The isolated report of gynecomastia in three male marihuana users generated considerable interest in the possibility that marihuana use could cause feminization. This report has not been corroborated but is still widely cited as evidence of such a possibility. In the context of undernutrition-related effects, it is of interest to note that gynecomastia has been noted during recovery from undernutrition. The fact that marihuana lacks estrogenic activity also make the possibility of feminization very unlikely.

Female reproductive function in animals has consistently been found to be adversely affected by cannabinoid administration. However, the female reproductive system is especially sensitive to undernutrition (Young, 1973; Zubiran & Gomez-Mont, 1953). For example, anestrus occurs in rats when body weight loss is only about 15% and ovarian atrophy, follicular atresia, and regression of corpora lutea are also related to undernutrition (Jackson, 1925). An unequivocal interpretation of marihuana's chronic effects on female reproductive function can only be arrived at after the nutritional issue has been properly dealt with.

On the other hand, studies of acute administration of cannabinoids very often yield results which are similar to those reported in chronic studies. In such cases it is unlikely that the results are due to secondary actions of drug administration such as decreased food and water consumption. Effects of cannabinoid administration on prolactin levels, for example, are quite consistent and this effect appears to be due to the pharmacological effects of marihuana. Moreover, this effect appears to have biological significance since lactation appears to be adversely affected by cannabinoids and this effect may be mediated by marihuana's inhibition of prolactin's actions.

References

Abel, E. L. Cannabis: Effects on hunger and thirst. *Behavior Biology*, 1975, *15*, 255.

Abel, E. L. *Marihuana: The first twelve thousand years.* Plenum Press, New York, 1980a.

Abel, E. L. A review of alcohol's effects on sex and reproduction. *Drug and Alcohol Dependence*, 1980b, *5*, 321.

Aldrich, M. R. Tantric cannabis use in India. *Journal of Psychedelic Drugs*, 1977, *9*, 137.

Asch, R. H., Fernandez, E. O., Smith, C. G., and Pauerstein, C. J. Precoital single doses of delta-9-tetrahydrocoannabinol block ovulation in the rabbit. *Fertility and Sterility*, 1979, *31*, 311.

Ayalon, D., Nir, I., Cordova, T., Bauminger,S., Puder, M., Naor, Z., Kashi, R., Zor, U., Harell, A., and Lindner, H. R. Acute effect of delta-1-tetrahydrocannabinol on the hypothalamo-pituitary-ovarian axis in the rat. *Neuroendocrinology*, 1977, *23*, 31.

Besch, N. F., Smith, C. G., Besch, P. K., and Kaufman, R. H. The effect of marihuana (delta-9-tetrahydrocannabinol) on the secretion of luteinizing hormone in the ovariectomized rhesus monkey. *American Journal of Obstetrics and Gynecology*, 1977, *128*, 635.

Bloomquist, E. R. *Marihuana*, Gencoe Press, Beverly Hills, California, 1968.

Bose, B. C., Saifi, A. Q., and Bhagwat, A. W. Effect of Cannabis Indica on hexobarbital sleeping time and tissue respiration of rat brain. *Archives of Internationales de Pharmacodynamic et de Therapie*, 1963, *141*, 520.

Bromley, B. L., Rabii, J., Gordon, J. H., and Zimmerman, E. Delta-9-tetrahydrocannabinol inhibition of suckling-induced prolactin release in the lactating rat. *Endocrinology and Research Communications*, 1978, *5*, 271.

Brown, J. *Cannabis indica;* A valuable remedy in menorrhagia. *British Medical Journal*, 1883, *1*, 1002.

Burstein, S. and Raz, A. Inhibition of prostaglandin E2 biosynthesis by delta-1-tetrahydrocannabinol. *Prostaglandins*, 1972, *2*, 369.

Burstein, S., Hunter, S. A., and Shoupe, T. S. Cannabinoid inhibition of rat luteal cell progesterone synthesis. *Research Communications in Chemistry, Pathology and Pharmacology*, 1979, *24*, 413.

Cates, W. and Pope, J. N. Gynecomastia and cannabis smoking. *American Journal of Surgery*, 1977, *134*, 613.

Chakravarty, I., Shah, P. G., Sheth, A. R., and Ghosh, J. J. Mode of action of delta-9-tetrahydrocannabinol on hypothalamo-pituitary function in adult female rats. *Journal of Reproduction and Fertility*, 1979, *57*, 113.

Chakravarty, I., Sheth, A. R., and Ghosh, J. J. Effect of acute delta-9-tetrahydrocannabinol treatment on serum luteinizing hormone and prolactin levels in adult female rats. *Fertility and Sterility*, 1975, *26*, 947.

Chakravarty, I., Sengupta, D., Bhattacharya, P., and Ghosh, J. J. Effect of treatment with cannabis extract on the water and glycogen contents of the uterus in normal and estradiol-treated prepubertal rats. *Toxicology and Applied Pharmacology*, 1975, *34*, 513.

Collu, R., Letart, J., Leboeuf, G., and Ducharme, J. R. Endocrine effects of chronic administration of psychoactive drugs to prepuberal male rats. *Life Science*, 1975, *16*, 533.

Collu, R. Endocrine effects of chronic intraventricular administration of delta-9-tetrahydrocannabinol to prepuberal and adult male rats. *Life Science*, 1976, *18*, 223.

Cooper, C. R. *Here's to crime.* Little, Brown, Boston, 1937.

Corcoran, M. E., Amit, Z., Malsbury, C. W., and Daykin, S. Reduction in copulatory behavior of male rats following hashish injections. *Research Communications in Chemistry, Pathology and Pharmacology*, 1974, *7*, 779.

Cushman, P. Plasma testosterone levels in healthy male marihuana smokers. *American Journal of Drug and Alcohol Abuse*, 1975, *2*, 269.

Cutler, M. G., Mackintosh, J. H., and Chance, M. R. A. Cannabis resin and sexual behaviour in the laboratory mouse. *Psychopharmacologia*, 1975, *45*, 129.

Daley, J. D., Branda, L. A., Rosenfeld, J., and Younglai, E. V. Increase of serum prolactin in male rats by (−)-*trans*-delta-9-tetrahydrocannabinol. *Journal of Endocrinology*, 1974, *63*, 415.

Dalterio, S. L., Perinatal or adult exposure to cannabinoids alters male reproductive functions in mice. *Pharmacology, Biochemistry, and Behavior*, 1980, *12*, 143.

Dalterio, S., Bartke, A., and Burstein, S. Cannabinoids inhibit testosterone secretion by mouse testes in vitro. *Science*, 1977, *196*, 1472.

Dalterio, S., Bartke, A., Roberson, C., Waton, D., and Burstein, S. Direct and pituitary-mediated effects of delta-9-tetrahydrocannabinol and cannabinnol on the testis. *Pharmacology, Biochemistry, and Behavior*, 1978, *8*, 673.

Davidson, J. M. Hormones and reproductive behavior. In *Hormones and behavior*, S. Levine (ed.), Academic Press, New York, 1972, 63–103.

Dixit, V. P., Sharma, V. N., and Lohiya, M. K. The effect of chronically administered cannabis extract on the testicular function of mice. *European Journal of Pharmacology*, 1974, *26*, 111.

Dixit, V. P., and Lohiya, N. K. Effects of cannabis extract on the response of accessory sex organs of adult male mice to testosterone. *Indian Journal of Physiology and Pharmacology*, 1975, *19*, 98–100.

Dwarakanath, C. Use of opium and *cannabis indica*, or Indian hemp. *Bulletin on Narcotics*, 1965, *17*, 15.

Fisher, G. and Steckler, A. Psychological effects, personality and behavioral changes attributed to marihuana use. *International Journal of the Addictions*, 1974, *9*, 101.

Freudenthal, R. I., Martin, J., and Wall, M. E. Distribution of delta-9-tetrahydrocannabinol in the mouse. *British Journal of Pharmacology*, 1972, *44*, 244.

Fujimoto, G. I., Kostellow, A. B., Rosenbaum, R., Morrill, G. A., and Bloch, E. Effects of cannabinoids on reproductive organs in the female fischer rat. In *Marihuana: biological effects*, G. G. Nahas and W. D. M. Patton (eds.), Pergamon Press, New York, 1979, 411.

Gay, G. R. and Sheppard, C. W. Sex-crazed dope fiends—Myth or reality? *Drug Forum*, 1973, *2*, 125.

Gay, G. R., Newmeyer, J. A., Elion, R. A., and Wieder, S. The sensuous hippie. Part 1: Drug/sex practice in the Haight-Ashbury. *Drug Forum*, 1977, *6*, 27.

Goode, E. Drug use and sexual activity on a college campus. *American Journal of Psychiatry*, 1972, *128*, 1272.

Gordon, J. H., Bromley, B. L., Gorski, R. A., and Zimmerman, E. Delta-9-tetrahydrocannabinol enhancement of lordosis behavior in estrogen-treated female rats. *Pharmacology, Biochemistry and Behavior*, 1978, *8*, 603.

Grigor, J. Indian hemp as an oxytocic. *Month. J. Med. Sci.*, 1852, *15*, 124.

Harmon, J. and Aliapoulios, M. A. Gynecomatia in marihuana users. *New England Journal of Medicine*, 1972, *287*, 936.

Harmon, J. W., Locke, D., Aliapoulios, M. A., and MacIndoe, J. H. Interference with testicular development of delta-9-tetrahydrocannabinol. *Surgical Forum*, 1976, *26*, 350.

Hembree, W. C., Zeidenberg, P., and Nahas, G. G. Marihuana's effects on human gonadal function. In *Marihuana: Chemistry, biochemistry and cellular effects*, G. G. Nahas (ed.), Springer Verlag, New York, 1976, 521.

Hembree, W. C., Nahas, G. G., Zeidenberg, P., and Huang, H. F. S. Changes in human spermatozoa associated with high dose marihuana smoking. In *Marihuana: Biological effects*, G. G. Nahas and W. D. M. Paton (eds.), Pergamon Press, Oxford, 1980, 429.

High times encyclopedia of recreational drugs. Stonehill Pub. Co., New York, 1978.

Hochman, J. S. and Brill, N. Qu. Chronic marihuana use and psychosocial adaptation. *American Journal of Psychiatry*, 1973, *130*, 132.

Huang, H. F. S., Nahas, G. G., and Hembree, W. C. Effects of marihuana inhalation on spermatogenesis of the rat. In *Marihuana: Biological effects*, G. G. Nahas and W. D. M. Paton (eds.), Pergamon Press, Oxford, 1980, 419.

Indian hemp drugs commission report. Gov't Printing Office, London, 1893–1894.

Issidorides, M. R. Observations in chronic hashish users: Nuclear observations in blood and sperm and abnormal acrosomes in spermatozoa. In *Marihuana: Bio-*

logical effects, G. G. Nahas and W. D. M. Paton (eds.), Pergamon Press, Oxford, 1980, 377.

Jackson, C. M. *The effects of inanition and malnutrition upon growth and structure.* P. Blakiston's Sons and Co., Philadelphia, 1925.

Jakubovic, A., McGeer, E. G., and McGeer, P. L. Effects of cannabinoids on testosterone and protein synthesis in rat testis Leydig cells in vitro. *Molecular and Cellular Endocrinol.*, 1979, 15, 41.

Kaestner, E., Rosen, L., and Appel, P. Patterns of drug abuse: Relationships with ethnicity, sensation seeking and anxiety. *Journal of Consulting and Clinical Psychology*, 1977, 45, 462.

Khavari, K. A., Humes, M., and Mabry, E. Personality correlates of hallucinogen use. *Journal of Abnormal Psychology*, 1977, 86, 172.

Koff, W. C. Marihuana and sexual activity. *Journal of Sex Research*, 1974, 10, 194.

Kolodny, R. C., Masters, W. H., Kolodner, R. M., and Toro, G. Depression of plasma testosterone levels after chronic intensive marihuana use. *New England Journal of Medicine*, 1974, 290, 872.

Kolodny, R. C., Lessin, P., Toro, G., Masters, W. H., and Cohen, J. Depression of plasma testosterone with acute marihuana administration. In *Pharmacology of Marihuana*, M. C. Braude and S. Szara (eds.), Raven Press, New York, 1976, 217.

Kolodny, R. C., Webster, S. K., Tullman, G. D., and Dornbush, R. I. Chronic marihuana use by women: Menstrual cycle and endocrine findings. Presented at New York University Postgraduate Medical School Second Annual Conference on Marihuana: Marihuana—Biomedical Effects and Social Implications, June 28–29, 1979.

Kramer, J. and Ben-David, M. Suppression of prolactin secretion by acute administration of delta-9-tetrahydrocannabinol in rats. *Proceedings of the Society of Experimental Biology and Medicine*, 1974, 147, 482.

Legator, M. S., Weber, E., Connor, T., and Stoeckel, M. Failure to detect mutagenic effects of delta-9-tetrahydrocannabinol in the dominant lethal test host-mediated assay, blood urine studies and cytogenic evaluation with mice. In *Pharmacology of Marihuana*, M. C. Braude and S. Szara (eds.), Raven Press, New York, 1976, 699.

Ley, W. Observations on the *Cannabis indica*, or Indian hemp. *Prov. Med. J. Retro. Med. Sci.*, 1843, 5, 487.

Ling, G. M., Thomas, J. A., Usher, D. R., and Singhal, R. L. Effects of chronically administered delta-1-tetrahydrocannabinol on adrenal and gonodal activity of male rats. *International Journal of Clinical Pharmacology*, 1973, 7, 1.

List, A., Nazar, S., Nyquist, S., and Harclerode, J. The effects of delta-9-tetrahydrocannabinol and cannabidiol on the metabolism of gonadal steroids in the rat. *Drug Metabolism and Disposition*, 1977, 5, 268.

Marks, B. H. Delta-1-tetrahydrocannabinol and luteinizing hormone secretion. *Progress in Brain Research*, 1973, 39, 331.

Maskarinec, M. P., Shipley, G., Novotny, M., Brown, D. J., and Forney, R. B. Different effects of synthetic delta-9-tetrahydrocannabinol and cannabis extract on steroid metabolism in male rats. *Experientia*, 1978, 34, 88–89.

Mendelson, J. H., Kuehnle, J., Ellingboe, J., and Babor, T. F. Plasma testosterone levels before, during, and after chronic marihuana smoking. *New England Journal of Medicine*, 1974, *291*, 1051.

Mendelson, J. H., Ellingboe, J., Kuehnle, J. C., and Mello, N. K. Effects of chronic marihuana use on integrated plasma testosterone and luteinizing hormone levels. *Journal of Pharmacology and Experimental Therapeutics*, 1978, *207*, 611.

Merari, A., Barak, A., and Plaves, M. Effects of delta-1(2)-tetrahydrocannabinol on copulation in the male rat. *Psychopharmacologia*, 1973, *28*, 243.

Mulinas, M. G. and Pomerantz, L. Pituitary replacement therapy in pseudohypophysectomy. *Endocrinology*, 1941, *29*, 558.

Nir, I., Ayalon, D., Tsafriri, A., Cordova, T., and Lindner, H. R. Suppression of the cyclic surge of luteinizing hormone secretion and of ovulation in the rat by delta-1-tetrahydrocannabinol. *Nature*, 1973, *243*, 470.

Okey, A. B. and Truant, G. S. Cannabis demasculinizes rats but is not estrogenic. *Life Science*, 1975, *17*, 1113.

Okey, A. B. and Bondy, G. P. Is delta-9-tetrahydrocannabinol estrogenic? *Science*, 1977, *195*, 904.

Okey, A. B. and Bondy, G. P. Delta-9-tetrahydrocannabinol and 17-beta-estradiol bind to different macromolecules in estrogen target tissues. *Science*, 1978, *200*, 312.

Purohit, V., Singh, H., and Ahluwalia, B. S. Evidence that the effects of methadone and marihuana on male reproductive organs are mediated at different sites on rats. *Biology of Reproduction*, 1979, *20*, 1039.

Raine, J. M., Wing, D. R., and Paton, W. D. M. The effects of delta-1-tetrahydrocannabinol on mammary gland growth, enzyme activity, and plasma prolactin levels in the mouse. *European Journal of Pharmacology*, 1978, *51*, 11.

Rawitch, A. B., Shultz, G. S., Ebner, K. E., and Vardaris, R. M. Competition of delta-9-tetrahydrocannabinol with estrogen in rat uterine estrogen receptor binding. *Science*, 1977, *197*, 1189.

Rose, R. M. Background paper on testosterone and marihuana. In *Marihuana and health hazards: Methodological issues in current research*, J. R. Tinklenberg (ed.), Academic Press, New York, 1975, 63.

Rosenkrantz, H., Heyman, I. A., and Braude, M. C. Inhalation, parenteral and oral LD50 values of delta-9-tetrahydrocannabinol in fischer rats. *Toxicology and Applied Pharmacology*, 1974, *28*, 18.

Rosenkrantz, H., Sprague, R. A., Fleischman, R. W., and Braude, M. C. Oral delta-9-tetrahydrocannabinol toxicity in rats treated for periods up to six months. *Toxicology and Applied Pharmacology*, 1975, *32*, 399.

Rosenkrantz, H. and Hayden, D. W. Acute and subacute inhalation toxicity of Turkish marihuana, cannabichromene, and cannabidiol in rats. *Toxicology and Applied Pharmacology*, 1979, *48*, 375.

Sassenrath, E. N. and Chapmen, L. F. Tetrahydrocannabinol-induced manifestations of the "marihuana-syndrome" in group-living macaques. *Federation Proceedings*, 1975, *34*, 1666.

Schaefer, C. F., Gunn, C. G., and Dubowski, K. M. Normal plasma testosterone concentrations after marihuana smoking. *New England Journal of Medicine*, 1975, *292*, 867.

Shoemaker, R. H. and Harmon, J. W. Suggested mechanism for demasculinizing effects of marihuana. *Federation Proceedings*, 1977, *36*, 345.

Smith, C. G., Besch, M., Smith, R. G., and Besch, P. K. Effect of tetrahydrocannabinol on the hypothalamic-pituitary axis in the ovariectomized rhesus monkey. *Fertility and Sterility*, 1979, *31*, 335.

Smith, C. G., Smith, M. T., Besch, M. F., Smith, R. G., and Asch, R. H. Effect of delta-9-tetrahydrocannabinol (THC) on female reproductive function. In *Marihuana: Biological effects*, G. G. Nahas and W. D. M. Paton (eds.), Pergamon Press, Oxford, 1980, 449.

Solomon, J., Cocchia, R., Gray, D., Shattuck, D., and Vossmer, A. Uterotrophic effect of delta-9-tetrahydrocannabinol in ovariectomized rats. *Science*, 1976, *192*, 559.

Symons, A. M., Teale, J. D., and Marks, V. Effect of delta-9-tetrahydrocannabinol on the hypothalamic-pituitary-gonadal system in the maturing male rat. *Journal of Endocrinology*, 1976, *67*, 43P–44P.

Tart, C. T. *On being stoned*. Science and Behavior Books, Palo Alto, California, 1971.

Thompson, G. R., Mason, M. M., Rosenkrantz, H., and Braude, M. C. Chronic oral toxicity of cannabinoids in rats. *Toxicology and Applied Pharmacology*, 1973, *25*, 373.

Thompson, G. R., Fleishman, R. W., Rosenkrantz, H., and Braude, M. C. Oral and intravenous toxicity of delta-9-tetrahydrocannabinol in rhesus monkeys. *Toxicology and Applied Pharmacology*, 1974, *27*, 648.

Traub, S. H. Perceptions of marijuana and its effects: A comparison of users and nonusers. *British Journal of Addiction*, 1977, *72*, 67.

Turley, W. A. and Floody, O. R. Delta-9-tetrahydrocannabinol stimulates receptive and proceptive sexual behaviors in female hamsters. *Pharmacology, Biochemistry, and Behavior*, 1981, *14*, 745.

Tyrey, L. Delta-9-tetrahydrocannabinol suppression of episodic luteinizing hormone secretion in the ovariectomized rat. *Endocrinology*, 1978, *102*, 1808.

Uyeno, E. T. Effects of delta-9-tetrahydrocannabinol and 2,5-dimethoxy-4-methylamphetamine on rat sexual dominance behavior. *Proceedings of the Western Pharmacological Society*, 1976, *19*, 369.

Virgo, B. B. The estrogenicity of delta-9-tetrahydrocannabinol (THC): THC neither blocks nor induces ovum implantation, nor does it effect uterine growth. *Research Communications in Chemistry, Pathology and Pharmacology*, 1979, *25*, 65.

Vyas, D. K. and Singh, R. Effect of cannabis and opium on the testis of the pigeon. *Columba Livia Gmelin Indian Journal of Experimental Biology*, 1976, *14*, 22.

Wilson, E. Crazy dreamers. *Collier's*, 1949, *123*, 27.

Wilson, G. T. and Lawson, D. M. Effects of alcohol on sexual arousal in women. *Journal of Abnormal Psychology*, 1976a, *85*, 489.

Wilson, G. T. and Lawson, D. M. Expectancies, alcohol, and sexual arousal in male social drinkers. *Journal of Abnormal Psychology*, 1976b, *85*, 587.

Young, W. C. (ed.), *Sex and internal secretions*, R. E. Krieger, Huntington, New York, 1973.

Zimmerman, A. M., Zimmerman, S., and Raj, A. Y. Effects of cannabinoids on spermatogenesis in mice. In *Marihuana: Biological effects*, G. G. Nahas and W. D. P. Paton (eds.), Permagon Press, Oxford, 1980, 407.

Zimmerman, Bruce, W. R. and Zimmerman, S. Effects of cannabinoids on sperm morphology. *Pharmacology*, 1979, *18*, 143.

Zubiran, S. and Gomez-Mont, F. Endocrine disturbances in chronic malnutrition. *Vitamins and Hormones*, 1953, *11*, 97.

Chapter 12

Methaqualone

Methaqualone was introduced into the United States in the 1960s as a nonbarbiturate sedative/hypnotic. Although originally considered to have low potential for abuse, methaqualone quickly gained the reputation of producing a "high" without also producing sedation and thereafter nontherapeutic usage became widespread.

At low doses (about 75 mg) the drug produces relaxation and tranquility. Adverse effects include fatigue, dizziness, headache, and numbness or tingling in the extremities. After moderate doses (about 200 mg), euphoria and self-confidence, followed by sedation, occur. With higher doses (400 mg), marked sedation occurs. Adverse effects at this dose include muscle weakness, delirium, tremor, agitation, panic, and respiratory depression.

Tolerance and physical dependence can both occur. Withdrawal is similar to that occurring in connection with barbiturate withdrawal.

Methaqualone is known as the "love drug" and "heroin for lovers." The terms indicate its reputation as an aphrodiasiac, and it has a widespread reputation in this context (e.g., Kramer, 1973; Inaba *et al.*, 1973; Kochansky *et al.*, 1975; Falco, 1976). However, Hollister (1976) comments that there are no reports by individuals who have taken the drug as a prescription sedative-hypnotic experiencing such effects.

Inaba and his co-workers (1973) note that as a sedative-hypnotic methaqualone is more likely to have a depressant effect on sexual function. Its reputation as an aphrodiasiac may thus be due to a lowering of inhibitions associated with depressant drugs in general.

MALE SEXUALITY

Anecdotal Evidence

Despite the one patient quoted by Inaba *et al.* (1973), most anecdotal comments about methaqualone tend to stress its positive effects with regard to sex. However, in many instances, the effect is on "set" rather than performance as noted by Inaba and co-workers. For example, Parr (1976) quotes a female user as stating: "(Methaqualone) heightens sex and relaxes you, so much that it breaks down inhibitions. It brings libido to the surface."

In contrast to this sentiment, however, Inaba and co-workers (1973) quote one of their patients as stating that: "(after taking methaqualone) I never got off, and it's also hard to get it up." Gay *et al.* (1977) likewise quote one of their clients to the effect that: "Methaqualone is a 'cheap thrill.' It ain't nothin' more than an over-publicized, over-rated, and over-glamourized 'red'."

In a later study, however, Gay and co-workers (1982) noted that methaqualone is often used to reduce inhibitions, especially in nontraditional settings such as homosexual liasons and group sex: "Ludes are best for anal sex. They let me pass out and I don't care." "When it comes to three-ways or multiple partners, consecutively, ludes keep you hard."

SURVEY STUDIES

Several survey studies have been reported in which respondents rated their preferences for methaqualone in connection with sexual activity.

Gerald and Schwirian (1973) surveyed 66 college students. Seventy-seven percent of those sampled stated that they expected the drug would increase libido and 97% stated they experienced this effect. Forty-two percent also stated that they expected the drug would reduce sexual inhibitions and 95% claimed it actually did so.

Kochansky and co-workers (1975) also surveyed college students (N=25) with respect to use of methaqualone and other drugs. All of the women surveyed stated a preference for methaqualone whereas the men surveyed expressed a preference for marihuana. Ten of the twelve students who responded to questions regarding methaqualone and sex stated it definitely increased sexual arousal and several stated using it for purposes of sexual seduction.

Parr (1976) surveyed 22 drug users attending a Drug Dependence Clinic in England. As in the Kochansky study, women preferred methaqualone over marihuana, whereas men rated marihuana first. Women also differed from men in this respect when asked about the effects of these drugs on libido and subjective sexual experience.

In their survey of drug users attending the Haight-Ashbury Free Medical Clinic and the Heroin Detoxification Clinic (Gay *et al.*, 1977), methaqualone was not used to any great extent "to make sex better" and was rated as similar to heroin in reducing sexual performance.

In their subsequent study of heterosexual, homosexual, and bisexual drug users, Gay *et al.* (1982) noted that methaqualone was cited by more than a third of the respondents overall as being used to enhance sex. Female heterosexuals and bisexuals rated it higher in this regard than their male counterparts, whereas the opposite was so for homosexual men and women. However, methaqualone was rated identically with alcohol in terms of increasing sexual pleasure and both were rated as only slightly positive in this regard. Again, women rated methaqualone higher with respect to increasing sexual pleasure than men. Lesbian women, in fact, rated methaqualone relatively high in this respect.

STUDIES IN ANIMALS

There are only two studies in which methaqualone's effects on sexual behavior have been reported (Claus *et al.*, 1980; 1981). In the first study, an injection of 10 mg/kg to a male monkey in a colony produced a transient increase in sexual behavior consisting of masturbation or autofellatio, but not copulation. In the second study, all animals in the colony were injected. This resulted in increased sexual arousal (penile erection), increased male–female contact, and copulatory behavior on the part of a male that had never previously engaged in such behavior.

SUMMARY AND CONCLUSIONS

There is little evidence in the human literature that methaqualone increases libido or affects sexual function. Studies in animals, however, do suggest that the drug increases sexual arousal.

References

Claus, G., Kling, A., and Bolander, K. Effects of methaqualone on social behavior in monkeys (Macaca Mulatta). *Brain Behavior Evolution*, 1980, *17*, 391–410.

Claus, G., Kling, A., and Bolander, K. Effects of methaqualone on social-sexual behavior in monkeys (M. Mulatta). *Brain Behavior Evolution*, 1981, *18*, 105–113.

Falco, M. Methaqualone misuse: Foreign experience and United States drug control policy. *International Journal of the Addictions*, 1976, *11*, 597–610.

Gay, G., Newmeyer, J., Elion, R., and Wieder, S. The sensous hippie Part I: Drug/Sex practice in the Haight-Ashbury. *Drug Forum*, 1977, *6*, 27–47.

Gay, G., Newmeyer, J. Perry, M. Johnson, G., and Kurland, M. Love and Haight: The sensuous hippie revisited. Drug/sex practices in San Francisco, 1980–81. *Journal of Psychoactive Drugs*, 1982, *14*, 111–123.

Gerald, M. C., Schwirian, P. M. Nonmedical use of methaqualone. *Archives of General Psychiatry*, 1973, *28*, 627–631.

Hollister, L. E. Minireview: Drugs and sexual behavior in man. *Life Sciences*, 1976, *17*, 661–668.

Inaba, D. S., Gay, G. R., Newmeyer, J. A., and Whitehead, C. Methaqualone abuse, "luding out." *Journal of the American Medical Association*, 1973, *224*, 1505.

Kochansky, G. E., Hemenway, T. S., Salzman, C., and Shader, R. I. Methaqualone abusers: A preliminary survey of college students. *Diseases of the Nervous System*, 1975, *36*, 348–351.

Kramer, S. Methaqualone as aphrodisiac. *American Journal of Psychiatry*, 1973, *130*, 1044.

Parr, D. Sexual aspects of drug abuse in narcotic addicts. *Brit. Journal of Addiction*, 1976, *71*, 261–268.

Chapter 13

Narcotics

Narcotics such as morphine are derived from the opium poppy, *Papaver somniferum*. The opium poppy contains about 10 percent morphine and about 0.5 percent codeine. Morphine was isolated from opium in 1806. Heroin (diacetylmorphine) is a semisynthetic derivative of morphine produced in 1898 by slightly altering the chemical structure of morphine. This enabled it to pass into the brain much faster than an equivalent dose of morphine. Once in the brain, however, heroin is converted back into morphine. Methadone is a synthetic opiate with a potency somewhat similar to morphine, but it has a longer duration of action. Although used in the treatment of withdrawal from heroin, methadone also can produce dependence. The basis of "methadone maintenance" is the blockade of euphoria associated with heroin and the reduction in the craving for heroin which methadone produces.

Like alcohol and marihuana, opium is one of the oldest psychoactive agents used by man. Descriptions of its behavioral effects can be traced as far back as 4000 B.C. These drugs produce a variety of effects including analgesia, sedation, euphoria or dysphoria, and respiratory depression. Nonmedical use is due to the euphoric sensation these drugs produce. Death due to overdosing arises from the respiratory depression produced by these drugs.

Tolerance and physical dependence develop rapidly to them. Withdrawal is characterized by symptoms similar to the flu, e.g., fever, chills, sweating, diarrhea.

Narcotic drugs are poorly absorbed from the stomach and intestine and therefore these drugs are usually not taken by mouth. Instead, they are injected either intramuscularly, subcutaneously, or intravenously. Sometimes they are also sniffed through a straw or they are burnt and the smoke is inhaled.

Although the brain is the main site of action of these drugs, only small amounts actually pass into the brain. Larger amounts are metabolized in the liver and excreted by the kidney. In the brain, narcotic drugs interact with specific receptors. These receptors are located throughout the brain but are mostly concentrated in the area of the limbic system, hypothalamus, thalamus, and spinal cord. Apparently, narcotic drugs resemble naturally occurring substances in the brain called endorphins and enkephalins which act like neurotransmitters. Narcotic drugs thus produce some of their effects by mimicking the actions of these endogenous neurochemicals. Narcotic drugs also inhibit the release of neurotransmitters such as dopamine, norepinephrine, and acetylcholine from presynaptic terminals. Although the pain-reducing properties of these drugs are believed to be due to their actions at receptors sites, the mechanism by which they affect mood and produce their other effects is still uncertain.

One common impression of the life-style of the "dope fiend" narcotic user is that of unbridled sexual orgies and barbarous sexual practices (Mathis, 1970). This impression, however, is the antithesis of clinical observations and studies.

MALE SEXUALITY

Anecdotal Reports

Anecdotal reports of male narcotics users about sexual activity generally note a decreased interest in sex coupled with an ability to prolong intercourse. For example, Burroughs (1953, p. 106) writes:

"Junk short-circuits sex. The drive to non-sexual sociability comes from the same place sex comes from, so when I have an H(eroin) or M(orphine) shooting habit I am non-sociable. If someone wants to talk, o.k. But there is no drive to become acquainted."

Larner (1967) quotes another narcotics user's experiences in this regard as follows:

"My sex drive, before narcotics, was so great that upon intercourse with a girl, I would achieve climax almost immediately. And I noticed something. That upon taking narcotics, it lulled my sex drive. But, on drugs, I was able to have sex for three, four hours at a time. Which made me feel superior over the girl. The girl was always begging me to stop, she couldn't take it, when it used to be the other way around, when I used to tell the girl, you're wearing me out, honey. I never reach a climax when I'm under the influence of narcotics, but mentally, I feel that I can satisfy the women I'm with" (p. 109).

Survey Studies and Clinical Reports

Several surveys and clinical studies of heroin and morphine users have reliably noted that use of such drugs can cause loss of sex drive, penile impotence, delayed ejaculation, and failure to achieve orgasm (see Table 13).

Gay and Sheppard (1973) interviewed 50 patients at the Haight-Ashbury Free Medical Clinic about drug usage and sex. Most of the respondents had come to the clinic for detoxification from heroin. Heroin was regarded as the drug which decreased libido and potency more than all others for which choices were available, e.g., alcohol, marihuana, amphetamines, barbiturates, hallucinogens, etc.

In a second study by this group (Gay et al., 1977), 95 patients at the same clinic were surveyed. Heroin was cited as the drug most likely to reduce libido, most likely to prevent orgasm, and most likely to cause impotence. On the other hand, heroin was the drug of choice if offered the alternative of sex versus drug use. This latter choice is in keeping with the autoerotic nature of heroin use (see below). In their most recent study, Gay et al. (1982) again found that both men and women regarded heroin as a drug which decreased sexual pleasure.

TABLE 13. Effects of Narcotics on Libido and Sexual Function

Reference	N	Drug	Failure to achieve orgasm	Failure to achieve erection	Loss of sex drive	Delayed or failed ejaculation
Hanbury et al. (1977)	50	Methadone	88%	50%	38%	15%
		Heroin	69%	44%	38%	6%
		Drug-free	6%	6%	0%	6%
Bloom & Butcher (1979)	179	Methadone		22%,22%,26%[a]		59%,51%,51%[a]
		Heroin		31%,21%,23%		56%,36%,44%
Espejo et al. (1973)	25	Methadone	50%	60%	60%	50%
Cushman (1972)	53	Heroin		49%	66%	68%
Smith et al. (1982)	42	Heroin		28%[b]	59%[b]	52%[b]
				2%[c]	2%[c]	2%[c]
Cicero et al. (1977b)	16	Heroin			100%	
	29	Methadone			96.5%	

[a]Divided into different age groups.
[b]Post-heroin use.
[c]Pre-heroin use.

As part of the Sexual Concerns and Substance Abuse Project, a training and education project connected with the Haight-Ashbury Medical Clinic and Institute for the Advanced Study of Human Sexuality, Smith *et al.* (1982) summarized their clinical experiences with 500 patients, which included social-sexual functioning prior to, during, and after heroin use. Early stages of heroin use were associated with improved sexual functioning characterized by delayed ejaculation and ability to sustain erection. [This effect on ejaculation may be one of the reasons opiates were regarded as aphrodisiacs.] However, for most of those describing such improvement, sexual dysfunction (primarily premature ejaculation) was present prior to drug use. Escalation of heroin use, however, was associated with decreased libido, impotence, and ejaculatory failure. During abstinence, sexual dysfunction continued for many, but was found to be a secondary effect due to poor social interactive skills. Heroin, in such cases, was resorted to for disinhibition and relaxation in sociosexual situations (cf. also Hanbury *et al.*, 1977).

Methadone maintenance is also commonly associated with sexual disorders (e.g., Martin *et al.*, 1973). Espejo *et al.* (1973) have noted that "interference with normal sexual function is considered to be one of the most aggravating side effects of methadone maintenance therapy." Likewise, Garbutt and Goldstein (1972) relate that "a majority of patients who left (a methadone maintenance treatment program) voluntarily cited the loss of sexual ability as a major reason for withdrawing."

Naltrexone, a narcotic antagonist, had an opposite effect on sexual functioning in 3 out of 8 men who had no previous history of narcotic use. The drug produced recurrent spontaneous erections in these men with penile erection occurring 1–3 hours after administration. This effect did not occur after placebo administration (Mendelson *et al.*, 1979). Naloxone, on the other hand, had no effect on sexual arousal, penile erection, or orgasm in a double blind study involving one male subject (Goldstein & Hansteen, 1977).

Studies in Animals

Morphine decreased sexual behavior in monkeys (Crowley *et al.*, 1974) and rats (McIntosh *et al.*, 1980).

Sexual behavior in male monkeys was not affected by methadone, naloxone, or naltrexone (Abbott *et al.*, 1980; Crowley *et al.*, 1975; Glick *et al.*, 1982). However, Braude and Morrison (1976) reported that naltrexone produced a dose-related increase in penile erection in monkeys during the early weeks of a one-year program of chronic administration. In contrast to the absence of effects on sexual behavior in monkeys, naloxone and naltrexone increased sexual behavior in rats (Myers & Baum, 1979; McIntosh *et al.*, 1980; Gessa *et al.*, 1979). Gessa *et al.* (1979) noted that this effect also occurred in sexually inactive males.

In male hamsters, methadone decreased sexual behavior without affecting general activity, and increased ejaculatory latency (Murphy, 1981b).

Several studies have investigated the role of endogenous opioids on sexual behavior. Myerson and Terenius (1977) reported that 1 μg of β-endorphin significantly reduced copulatory behavior in male rats without affecting their motor activity. This effect was reversed by naltrexone. Pellegrini Quarantotti *et al.* (1978) reported that intraventricular injection of 6 μg of the enkephalen analog (D-Ala)-met-enkephalinamide also completely suppressed copulatory behavior in rats without affecting motor activity. This suppression was abolished by naloxone. McIntosh *et al.* (1980) reported that β-endorphin eliminated sexual behavior in male rats without affecting their general motor activity. Prior treatment with naloxone (30 mg/kg) prevented these inhibitory effects.

In summary, anecdotal reports, surveys, clinical reports in humans, and studies in animals agree that narcotic drugs and endogenous opioids exert an inhibitory effect on male sexual behavior and function, whereas narcotic antagonists may stimulate such behavior and function.

Effects on Sperm and Reproductive Organs

Sperm counts were not initially different among heroin, methadone, and non-narcotic users after two days of sexual abstinence. After sexual abstinence of three days or more, sperm counts were significantly higher among methadone users compared to controls (Cicero *et al.*, 1975). Heroin users had higher sperm counts than controls after sexual abstinence, but differences were not statistically significant. Sperm motility, on the other hand, was considerably lower among heroin and methadone users compared to controls. Ejaculated volume was lower in methadone and heroin users (Cicero *et al.*, 1975). These observations are in keeping with reports in animals of narcotics-induced effects on seminal vesicles (see below). These data also suggest methadone reduces male fertility more than heroin. In this regard Cicero *et al.* (1975) point out that although men on a methadone maintenance program did not father any children while participating in the program, they had fathered 53 children beforehand. Heroin users, on the other hand, remained fertile as indicated by the number of children fathered.

Studies in Animals

Three days of continuous exposure to morphine (75 mg) produced a significant decrease in prostate and seminal vesicle weights but not in testes weights in rats, relative to controls (Cicero *et al.*, 1974, 1975). Methadone (20 mg/kg) likewise produced a dose-related decrease in testes weight, seminal vesicle weight, and prostate weight in mice after chronic treatment for 5 days. When administered for 10 days, testes and prostate weights were reduced even further (Thomas & Dombrosky, 1975).

A decrease in testes weight produced by morphine was associated with a marked decrease in visible secretory vacuoles in seminal vesicles (Cicero *et al.*, 1975). The absence of associated degenerated necrotic cells indicated that the decreased weight of seminal vesicles was due to a reduction in cellular size and secretory content rather than a decrease in cell number (Cicero *et al.*, 1975). Cessation of morphine treatment resulted in a return to control weight by the seventh day of abstinence (Cicero *et al.*, 1974). Differences in body weight or water intake between drug-treated animals and controls was minimal suggesting that the observed differences were not due to nutritional factors (Cicero *et al.*, 1974).

Chronic methadone and morphine administration increased the incidence of dominant lethal mutations in mice. The increase was correlated with an increase in observable incidence of chromosomal abnormalities in sperm (Badr *et al.*, 1979).

These clinical and experimental studies indicate that narcotic drugs adversely affect male fertility. This effect appears greater for heroin than methadone, but does not appear to be irreversible.

EFFECTS ON HORMONES

Testosterone

Most studies have noted decreased serum testosterone levels in narcotics users (see Table 14). The major exception are the studies by Cushman (1972, 1973). Since many of these studies involved outpatients, differences in results could have been due to several factors such as difficulties in evaluating histories (generally unreliable), differences in dosage taken by users (impure heroin of varying amounts), differences in time between drug taken and blood sampling, individual differences in episodic secretory hormonal patterns, and methodological problems in measuring hormonal levels (protein binding versus radioimmunoassay) (cf. Mirin *et al.*, 1976; Thomas *et al.*, 1977).

Many heroin users and methadone users also tend to consume large amounts of alcohol (Cushman, 1973). Conceivably, some of the reported changes in hormonal levels may be due more to alcohol consumption than narcotic usage (Abel, 1980). However, decreased testosterone levels were also noted in a group of heroin

TABLE 14. Effect of Narcotics on Testosterone Levels

Reference	Drug	Testosterone levels
Bolelli *et al.* (1979)	Heroin	↓
	Methadone	↓
Cicero *et al.* (1977b)	Heroin	↓
	Methadone	—
	Controls	
Cushman (1972)	Heroin	—
	Methadone	—
Cushman (1973)	Methadone	—
	Heroin	—
	Controls	
Cushman (1973)	Methadone	—
Lafisca *et al.* (1981)	Methadone (30 mg/day)	—
Mendelson *et al.* (1975a)	Heroin	↓
	Methadone (80–150 mg/day)	↓
	Methadone (10–60 mg/day)	—
	Controls	
Mendelson *et al.* (1975a)	Methadone	↓
	Heroin	↓
Mendelson *et al.* (1980)	Heroin	↓
Mendelson & Mello (1975)	Heroin	↓
	Methadone	↓

users in Hong Kong where alcohol use is minimal (Mendelson and Mello, 1975).

In a clinical setting wherein many of the problems noted above were controlled, Mirin *et al.* (1976) administered heroin (10 mg) intravenously to 2 former heroin users. Testosterone levels did not decrease until about 4–6 hours after drug administration. Naltrexone administration prior to heroin reversed the decrease in testosterone levels.

In a similar study, Mendelson *et al.* (1975c; 1980) obtained daily blood samples from 10 previous heroin users prior to, and during 10 days of self-administration, followed by methadone maintenance. Testosterone levels fell significantly during methadone exposure compared to the drug-free period. Significant decreases in testosterone did not occur until 2.5 to 5 hours after heroin exposure. After cessation of methadone, testosterone levels increased to pre-heroin levels. In a second study, Mendelson *et al.* (1975a) reported that heroin addicts maintained on high dosages of methadone (80–150 mg/day) had depressed levels of testosterone, whereas testosterone levels in those receiving low dosage methadone (10–60 mg/day) did not differ from levels in nondrug-using controls. Testosterone levels were not lower after chronic heroin usage (10 mg, i.v./day) compared to acute exposure, suggesting possible tolerance to heroin's effects on testosterone or compensating gonadal steroid feedback (Mendelson *et al.*, 1980).

Animal Studies

Morphine reliably decreased testosterone levels in rats (e.g., Cicero *et al.*, 1974, 1975, 1976, 1977b). A single injection of morphine (20 mg/kg) had no effect on serum testosterone levels in rats up to one hour after injection. By two hours after injection, levels were significantly depressed. Maximum depression to about 85% of control levels occurred at four hours after injection. Levels returned to normal at seven hours postinjection, and by eight hours postinjection, levels were increased significantly compared to controls (Cicero *et al.*, 1976). Tolerance to morphine's effects on testosterone began to occur by about 11 days after chronic exposure and levels returned to normal by 20 days after exposure in rats (Cicero *et al.*, 1976).

Naloxone is able to antagonize the effects of morphine on testosterone levels, suggesting specificity of narcotics on testosterone (Cicero *et al.*, 1976). Further indication of the specificity of narcotic drugs on testosterone is evident from the greater potency of (−) narcotic isomers than (+) narcotic isomers. Methadone has about one-half the potency of morphine on testosterone levels (Cicero *et al.*, 1976).

Luteinizing and Follicle Stimulating Hormones

Data on the effect of narcotics on luteinizing hormone levels have not been consistent. No differences in LH levels between active heroin users, abstinent heroin users, methadone users, and controls have been reported in several studies (see Table 15). Although Martin *et al.* (1973) and Lafisca *et al.* (1981) reported decreases in LH associated with methadone administration, the decreased levels were still within clinically-normal levels.

Under controlled laboratory conditions, Mirin *et al.* (1976) reported that infusion of heroin (10 mg) produced a significant decrease in LH levels, but did not alter FSH levels in two detoxified male heroin users. This decrease was blocked by the administration of naltrexone. Naltrexone alone caused an increase in episodic LH release.

In a similar clinical setting, Mendelson *et al.* (1980) reported that acute doses of heroin (10 mg, i.v.) reduced LH levels in heroin users prior to pre-drug use levels. Chronic heroin use for 10 days did not produce any greater decrease in LH than initial exposure, indicating tolerance. Cessation of heroin use resulted in an increase in LH levels. Naltrexone produced an increase in LH levels in men with prior narcotics use (Mendelson *et al.*, 1979), and an even greater increase in LH in heroin users (Mendelson *et al.*, 1980), indicating possible "supersensitivity" of the hypothalamic-pituitary-gonadal axis during abstinence. Such supersensitivity has

TABLE 15. Effects of Narcotics on LH and FSH in Men

Reference	Drug	LH	FSH
Lafisca *et al.* (1981)	Methadone	↓	↓
Martin *et al.* (1973)	Methadone	↓	↓
Cushman (1972)	Heroin	—	
	Methadone	—	
Cushman (1973)	Methadone	—	—
Cushman (1973)	Methadone	—	
Azizi *et al.* (1973)	Heroin	—	—
	Methadone	—	—
Mendelson, Ellingboe, Kuehnle, & Mello (1980a)	Heroin	↓	
	Naltrexone	↑	
Bolelli *et al.* (1979)	Heroin	—	—
Mirin *et al.* (1976)	Heroin	↓	—
	Naltrexone	↑	

been reported in animals chronically treated with narcotics by Cicero *et al.* (1983).

Cicero *et al.* (1976) reported that a single administration of 20 mg/kg of morphine produced a significant decrease in LH levels in rats by 1 hour after administration. Levels remained reduced 25–50% for 1–5 hours and returned to normal by 6–8 hours. Depression in serum LH preceded depression of testosterone by about 1–2 hours (cf. also Cicero *et al.*, 1977a,b). The effects of morphine on LH were inhibited by naloxone (Cicero *et al.*, 1977b) and tolerance to morphine's effects on LH developed by about 17 days after initial exposure (Cicero *et al.*, 1977b).

Prolactin

Relatively little attention has been focussed on narcotic effects on prolactin. Tolis *et al.* (1975) reported that morphine produced an increase in serum prolactin in women. Studies in animals are also quite consistent in noting an increase in serum prolactin levels following narcotics administration or endogenous opiate exposure (Bruni *et al.*, 1977; Ferland *et al.*, 1977; Gold *et al.*, 1979; Gold *et al.*, 1978; Mendelson *et al.*, 1980), whereas narcotic antagonists produce decreases in serum prolactin (Bruni *et al.*, 1977; Gold *et al.*, 1978, 1979), as does withdrawal (Lal *et al.*, 1977; Gold *et al.*, 1981) indicating the opioids have a modulatory role in prolactin secretion.

FEMALE REPRODUCTION

Currently, there are about 100,000 women dependent on narcotic drugs in the United States (Martin & Martin, 1980). This is about four times fewer users compared to male narcotic users (Martin & Martin, 1980). This ratio is considerably different from that which existed prior to passage of the Harrison Narcotic Act in 1914 when there were many more women (1.4–2.0 times) using narcotics than men (Terry & Pellens, 1928) because of the high opiate content of many of the patent medicines of that era routinely used for "female troubles."

Women who use narcotics still experience "female troubles"—problems in sexual physiology, along with problems in sexual activity. At issue is the question of whether narcotic drugs precipitate such problems or are taken to alleviate them.

Anecdotal Reports

In general, there has been fewer literary comments about the effects of narcotics on female libido and sexual performance than comparable comments for men. Those which have appeared corroborate the impression from the male perspective. For example, Hughes (1967, p. 128) describes her own inability to achieve orgasm after taking heroin: ". . . horse (heroin) does affect you sexually, in a lot of ways. I mean, for instance, it's almost impossible to have an orgasm beyond eight caps. It can be done but it's unusual."

Survey and Clinical Reports

Wielund and Yunger (1971) reported that out of 15 women they examined, 11 experienced decreased libido while using heroin. When these women were switched to methadone, 10 out of the 15 claimed an increase in libido. Sexual activity was also lowered during heroin use for 11 of these women. When these women switched to methadone, sexual activity remained decreased for only 5 of them. Enjoyment of sex also increased after switching to methadone for 5 to 8 of the 15 women studied.

Frigidity is increased among female narcotic users. Ellinwood *et al.* (1966) reported that 27% of the women studied at Lexington stated they were frigid "at all times," and 10% said they were frigid "with most men." Smith and co-workers (1982) reported that 47% of the heroin users they studied had sexual concerns prior to drug use and this increased to 58% after beginning heroin use.

Naloxone decreased hypersexuality in a woman with adrenal insufficiency. When naloxone treatment stopped, hypersexuality returned (Blum *et al.*, 1983). In a "double-blind" study involving three "sexually unresponsive women," naloxone failed to affect sexual arousal (Brady & Bianco, 1980).

Studies in Animals

With the exception of the study by Crowley and co-workers (1975) regarding methadone's effects on sexual behavior in monkeys, the effects of opiates on sexual behavior in female animals has not been reported. With respect to the Crowley *et al.* (1975) study, methadone did not affect the frequency of sexually-related behaviors.

Menstruation

Effects of narcotics on the menstrual cycle are summarized in Table 16. Stoffer (1968) reported that 7% of a group of 81 heroin users had abnormal menstrual cycles prior to heroin use, 90% had abnormalities during use, and 48% had abnormalities three months after use. Bai *et al.* (1974) reported a similarly high incidence (85%) of menstrual disorders among their sample of 40 heroin users.

Gaulden *et al.* (1964) reported that length of menstrual cycle was normal prior to heroin use, whereas during use, 64% of the 72 women studied had cycles of 35 days or longer or they experienced complete elimination of menstruation. Termination of heroin use resulted in a return to normal cycle length for most women.

Amenorrhea began, on the average, about 17 months after initiation of heroin use, with a range of 1–72 months among the heroin users monitored by Stoffer (1968). After withdrawal, menses returned about 1.8 months later, with a range of a few days to 12 months.

Litt and Cohen (1970) reported that amenorrhea began 2–8 months after onset of heroin use among 148 adolescent girls and

TABLE 16. Effects of Narcotics on Menstruation

Reference	Sample size (drug)	Amenor-rhea[a]	Oligomenor-rhea[b]	Hypomenor-rhea[c]	Hypomenor-rhea[c] and polymenor-rhea[d]	Polymenor-rhea[d]	Total incidence of menstrual disorders
Bai *et al.* (1974)	40 (Heroin)	45%	15%	7.5%		12%	85%
Stoffer (1968)	81 (Heroin)	63%	10%	9%	7%	1%	90%
Litt & Cohen (1970)	256 (Heroin)	21%					21%
Santen *et al.* (1975)	76 (Heroin & Methadone)						70%
Wallach *et al.* (1969)	83 (Heroin)						67%
	83 (Methadone)						1%
Wielund & Yunger (1970)	15 (Heroin)	53%	20%				73%
	15 (Methadone)	6.6%	6.6%		6.6%		20%
Gaulden *et al.* (1964)	72 (Heroin)	65%					65%

[a]Amenorrhea—Cessation of menses.
[b]Oligomenorrhea—Reduced frequency of menses (interval more than 38 days and less than 3 months).
[c]Hypomenorrhea—Reduction in duration and flow of menses.
[d]Polymenorrhea—Shortening of interval between menses (less than 20 days).

normal menses returned by about 2 months after cessation. Santen *et al.* (1975) reported that 95% of a group of 76 narcotics users (heroin or methadone) experienced normal menses prior to drug use, but after initiating drug use, normal menses was experienced by only 30% of these women.

Methadone users experience a lower incidence of amenorrhea and anovulation compared to heroin users. Wallach *et al.* (1969) reported that 67% of 83 heroin users had menstrual disorders. When these women were switched to methadone, only 1% continued to have irregular menstruation. A similar reduction in menstrual problems following a switch from heroin to methadone was noted by Wielund and Yunger (1971).

In summary, both heroin and methadone use are associated with decreased libido or decreased sexual activity in women as well as irregular menstrual function. In many reports, however, the relation of these disorders to drug use was not evaluated with respect to sequence, i.e., whether these disorders preceded or followed drug use. Heroin has a much greater impact on libido and menstrual function than methadone. The effects of both drugs on libido and menstruation are reversible and normal menstruation function returns within months of disuse of these drugs.

One reason that methadone users experience fewer menstrual problems than heroin users may be that methadone users are a select, rather than a random population. They are likely to have better nutritional status than heroin users and better overall medical care (Blatmen, 1973).

Effects on Hormones

There have been very few studies of the effects of narcotics on hormones in women. The few studies that have been done have noted that in methadone-related amenorrhea, cyclic changes in FSH were abolished (cf. also Bolelli *et al.*, 1979) and mid-cycle peaks in serum gonadotrophins and the luteal increases in serum progesterone also failed to occur (Santen *et al.*, 1975; cf also Bolelli *et al.*, 1979).

Morphine (10 mg) produced a significant rise (390%) in serum prolactin levels in a number of women tested just prior to elective gynecological survey (Tolis *et al.*, 1975). Naloxone was found to produce an increase in LH and FSH levels in nonopiate-using women with hyperprolactinemia (Grossman *et al.*, 1982). Reid *et al.* (1981) reported that intravenous administration of β-endorphin produced a small, but statistically significant, rise in LH in a group of women. Vrbicky *et al.* (1982) observed a statistically significant increase in β-endorphin levels two days prior to the LH surge, and a significant decrease in β-endorphin levels five days after the LH surge in a number of women. These observations suggest an involvement of opiate-mediated mechanisms in regulation of LH.

Studies in Animals

In animals, morphine at very high doses (35–60 mg/kg) blocked spontaneous ovulation (Barraclough & Sawyer, 1955; Marko & Romer, 1983; Packman & Rothchild, 1976; Pang *et al.*, 1974). Ovulation eventually returned following a long period of abstinence (Barraclough & Sawyer, 1955). Morphine's blockade of ovulation was reversed by naloxone (Packman & Rothchild, 1976).

Relatively low doses of morphine (10 mg/kg) increased LH levels (Pang *et al.*, 1974), whereas higher doses (60 mg/kg) decreased the preovulatory surge of LH (Pang *et al.*, 1974; Muraki *et al.*, 1977, 1979; Sylvester *et al.*, 1980). Naloxone did not affect proestrus surge of LH (Muraki *et al.*, 1977), but did reverse morphine's inhibitory effects on LH (Muraki *et al.*, 1977).

SITE OF HORMONAL ACTION

The principal site of action of narcotic drugs on testosterone and LH regulation appears to be located within the central nervous system, and specifically in the hypothalamus, rather than peripherally in the testes or pituitary. Evidence against direct action on the testes are: 1) narcotics do not affect basal production of testosterone or gonadotropin-stimulated release of testosterone from the testes *in vitro* (Cicero *et al.*, 1977b); 2) the decrease in testosterone levels associated with morphine administration occurs long after serum morphine levels have decreased (Cicero *et al.*, 1977b), indicating that morphine does not directly affect production, release, or metabolism of testosterone; and 3) morphine does not affect testosterone levels in male rats hypophysectomized and maintained on hCG. Also worth noting is that the action of narcotics on testosterone levels are very stereospecific (Cicero *et al.*, 1976), and these effects can be competitively inhibited by naloxone (Cicero *et al.*, 1976), all of which suggest the testes are not directly involved in the action of narcotics on testosterone.

Evidence against direct pituitary involvement is based on these observations: 1) acute and chronic administration of narcotics lower LH levels in contrast to the expected rise in LH that ought to occur due to the negative peripheral feedback relation between LH and testosterone (Cicero *et al.*, 1977b); 2) the effect of narcotics on LH is stereospecific (Cicero *et al.*, 1977b); 3) morphine does not affect pituitary content of LH or LH-RH-induced pituitary release of LH (Cicero *et al.*, 1977a); 4) endogenous opioids or naloxone do not affect pituitary LH release *in vitro* (Cicero *et al.*, 1979; Shaar *et al.*, 1977).

Evidence for a central site of action for the effects of narcotics on testosterone and LH regulation are: 1) similarity between the effects of narcotic drugs and endogenous opioids in depressing serum LH levels (Bruni *et al.*, 1977; Cicero *et al.*, 1979; Meites *et al.*, 1979); 2) the similarity in the antagonism of these suppressive effects on LH by narcotic antagonists (Bruni *et al.*, 1977); 3) the increase in serum LH levels in humans and animals produced by narcotic antagonists administered alone (Bruni *et al.*, 1977; Blank *et al.*, 1979; Cicero *et al.*, 1979; Cicero *et al.*, 1980; Mendelson *et al.*, 1979; Mirin *et al.*, 1976; Meites *et al.*, 1979; Muraki *et al.*, 1977); and 4) the reversal of testosterone's negative feedback effects on LH levels by naloxone (Cicero *et al.*, 1979).

Studies in animals have localized regulation of LH via LH-RH in the ventral and medial hypothalamus (Blake & Sawyer, 1974).

This area has also been found to contain numerous opiate receptor binding sites and high levels of endogenous opiate peptides (Snyder, 1975).

These observations suggest that opioid receptors are involved in regulation of the hypothalamic-pituitary-LH axis and that naturally occurring opioids normally exert a tonic inhibitory effect on this axis. Narcotic drugs produce a similar effect by mimicking the actions of naturally occurring opioids on LH-RH/LH release.

Hypothalamic regulation of testosterone may occur as a result of competition between narcotics and androgens for opioid receptors in the hypothalamus, or by affecting hypothalamic control of LH.

The possibility that narcotics affect testosterone by competing with androgens for hypothalamic-receptor sites is based on the fact that both testosterone and opiates are derivates for perhydrophenathene (Thomas *et al.*, 1977) and that, at high concentrations, narcotics displace ^{3}H-testosterone from binding sites in the liver (LaBelle, 1975). However, such competitive displacement does not occur in the brain or hypothalamus (LaBelle *et al.*, 1978; Cicero *et al.*, 1979a) making this possibility less viable.

MECHANISM OF ACTION

Explanations for the narcotics user's loss of libido and reproductive dysfunction fall into three main categories: 1) narcotics produce substitute sexual satisfaction—the psychoanalytical hypothesis; 2) effects on libido and reproduction are due to narcotics-related impaired health; 3) narcotics produce physiological changes which directly affect the neural mechanisms that control sexual function and behavior; and 4) effects are due to direct actions of narcotics on brain mechanisms that control these functions.

1. Psychoanalytical Interpretations

In 1926 Rado proposed a psychoanalytic basis for narcotics use which placed considerable emphasis on what he called the "phar-

macogenic" orgasm. According to Rado, injection of narcotics produces an erotic gratification which competes with natural sexual
gratification, and which has advantages over the latter. Some of
these advantages are that pharmacological orgasms can be
achieved without any need to interact with others and within seconds of injection. To Rado (1926) the pleasurable feeling of a full
stomach ("alimentary orgasm") resulting from narcotics use, cre-
ates a general diffused feeling of well-being which extends over the
whole body. Rado defined this sense of well-being as the goal of
sexual orgasm and argued that any means of such attainment
could become a substitute for actual sexual activity.

This concept was developed and refined in subsequent writings in the psychoanalytic literature (e.g., Fort, 1954; Wikler &
Rasor, 1953) and was traced to the oral level of sexual maturity in
conjunction with the state of bliss which the young infant experiences in receiving warm milk (cf. Smith *et al.*, 1982).

Systematic interviews of narcotics users corroborated the relation between drug use and alimentary sensations (Chessick, 1960).
Most users stated experiencing a warmth, usually localized in the
stomach and sometimes in the genitals. All reported a decrease in
sexual drive during the pharmacogenic orgasm.

Most recently, Tenhauten (1982) has once again attempted to
account for the decrease in sexual activity in terms of a psychoanalytic framework. The reason for the narcotics user's decreased
libido is that intravenous narcotics injection becomes a symbolic
sexual substitute for genital sexual activity. In this framework, the
narcotics user satisifes sexual needs symbolically (e.g., the needle
= penis). Narcotics use thereby becomes a substitute for sex, allowing the user to experience orgasm without sexual involvement
which might otherwise make him anxious due to personality
disturbance.

Although the link between narcotics use and alimentary satisfaction has been frequently noted, as has the symbolism of the
needle and the injection process, no experimental studies have
been directed at these interesting relationships.

2. Health and Nutritional Status

Narcotic usage is also frequently associated with health problems. Abnormal liver function occurs in about 80% of narcotic users. Primary problems include hepatitis and abnormal cell development. Lung disease is also present in about 95% of narcotic users. Cardiac disorders of various types occur in about 80% of narcotic users. Venereal disease occurs in about 60% of female narcotic users (Perlmutter, 1977).

Nutritonal status is often poor. Perlmutter (1977, p. 36) comments: "When dealing with drug addicts, one rarely sees an overweight or obese patient." Poor nutrition is usually found in conjunction with high carbohydrate intake when drug supplies are low and the narcotics users resort to sweets as a substitute. Recurrent and chronic disease places even greater demands on nutritional requirements (Perlmutter, 1977).

As early as 1925, Jackson noted how susceptible the female reproductive system was to weight loss. This relation has been documented in many reports (e.g., Young, 1973; Zubiran & Gomez-Mont, 1953). Inhibition of ovulation occurs in rats when body weight is decreased by only 15% and weight loss is associated with ovarian atrophy, follicular atresia, and regressing corpora lutea (Jackson, 1925; Young, 1973). The effects of narcotics on female menstrual function could thus be an indirect result of the effects of these drugs on nutritional status. Effects of undernutrition on males are more unreliable, however. In some cases, undernutrition is associated with testicular atrophy, but this is not always so (e.g., Mulinas & Pomerantz, 1941).

3. Hormonal Involvement

In conjunction with the decreases in levels of sex hormones produced by narcotics, one possible mechanism whereby narcotic drugs affect libido and sexual functioning is indirectly via their effect on hormonal secretion. This possibility is supported by the well-known relation between androgens, libido, and sexual function. For example, surgical castration is associated with decreased libido and erectile dysfunction (e.g., Luttge, 1971). Anti-androgen administration, the equivalent of chemical castration, likewise results in decreased libido and erectile dysfunction (Cooper & Ismail, 1972), whereas androgen replacement therapy can restore libido or sexual functioning in hypogonadal men (e.g., Luttge, 1971). However, normal testosterone levels have been found in adult males with impotence (Hudson & Coghlan, 1968), and sexual activity still occurs years after surgical castration in some men (Schiavi & White, 1976), and in hypogonadal men (Money & Ehrhardt, 1973). Thus, while androgens are undoubtedly involved in modulating libido and sexual activity, such activity is not solely dependent on changes in these hormones. On the other hand, the decrease in testes size and function associated with narcotics administration are probably due to suppression of testosterone which maintains the integrity and function of secondary sex organs (Mann, 1964). The difficulty in achieving erection and ejaculation associated with use of narcotics may be due to effects of these drugs on spinal-neural pathways mediating these effects. No direct studies have as yet been made of this possibility.

The effects of narcotics on testosterone and LH levels are due to the action of these drugs on the central nervous system rather than on peripheral sites such as the testes or pituitary. The mechanism may involve inhibition of ability to stimulate release of LH-RH via direct action on opioid receptors (see below).

4. Direct Effects on the Central Nervous System

None of the previous proposals is capable of accounting for the immediate suppressive effects of endogenous opioids or narcotic drugs on male sexual behavior or stimulation of such behavior by narcotic antagonists in animals. These studies in animals suggest that the reduction in sexual receptivity associated with narcotic drugs is due to a direct effect on central nervous system centers which control such receptivity, or on neurotransmitters which mediate such receptivity. Endogenous opioids have also been implicated in regulation of testosterone and LH activity where they appear to exert a tonic inhibitory effect. Narcotic drugs mimic this effect by stimulating the same receptors as those activated by the endogenous opioids.

Several studies have now suggested a close interaction between catecholamine-containing neurons and enkephalin-containing neurons (Palmer *et al.*, 1983). In this regard, the interplay between endogenous opioids and catecholamine levels and receptors (Palmer *et al.*, 1983) is especially of interest because of dopamine's reported involvement in male sexual behavior in rats (e.g., Tagliamonte *et al.*, 1973), and the andrenergic control of ejaculation (Kimura *et al.*, 1972). *In vitro* studies showing that morphine, metenkaphalen, and naloxone do not affect basal LH-RH release from the hypothalamus (Rotsztejn *et al.*, 1978a,b; Cicero *et al.*, 1979) whereas morphine and met-enkephalin inhibit dopamine-stimulated release of LH-RH (Rotsztejn *et al.*, 1978a,b), an effect which is abolished by naloxone (Rotsztejn *et al.*, 1978a,b), suggests that opiates modulate catecholamine-mediated nueronal activity underlying sexual function and physiology.

References

Abbott, O. A., Holman, S. D., and Goy, R. W. *Antagonists of brain opiates fail to stimulate the sexual behavior of the rhesus monkeys*. Paper presented at the Eastern Conference on Reproductive Behavior, New York, 1980.

Abel, E. A. A review of alcohol's effects on sex and reproduction. *Drug and Alcohol Dependence*, 1980, *5*, 321–332.

Azizi, F., Vagenakis, A. G., Longcope, C., Ingbar, S. H., and Braverman, L. E. Decreased serum testosterone concentration in male heroin and methadone addicts. *Steroids*, 1973, *22*, 467–472.

Badr, F. M., Rabouh, S. A.,and Badr, R. S. On the mutagenicity of methadone hydrochloride. *Mutation Research*, 1979, *68*, 235–249.

Bai, J., Greenwald, E., Caterini, H., and Kaminetzky, H. A. *Obstetrics and Gynecology*, 1974, *44*, 713–719.

Barraclough, C. A. and Sawyer, C. H. Inhibition of the release of pituitary ovulatory hormone in the rat by morphine. *Endocrinology*, 1955, *57*, 329–337.

Blake, C. A., Sawyer, C. H. Effects of hypothalamic deafferentiation on the pulsatile rhythm in plasma concentrations of luteinizing hormone in ovariectomized rats. *Endocrinology*, 1974, *94*, 730–736.

Blank, M. S., Panerai, A. E., and Friesen, H. G. Opioid peptides modulate luteinizing hormone secretion during sexual maturation. *Science*, 1979, *203*, 1129–1131.

Blatmen, S. Methadone effects on pregnancy and the newborn. *Proceedings Third National Conference on Methadone Treatment*, 1973, 842–845.

Bloom, W. A. and Butcher, B. T. Methadone side effects and related symptoms in 200 methadone maintenance patients. *Third National Conference on Methadone Treatment*, 1979, 44–47.

Blum, I., Elizur, A., Segal, A., Ochshorn, M., and Simantov, R. Effect of naloxone on the neuropsychiatric symptoms of a woman with partial 21-hydroxylase deficiency. *American Journal of Psychiatry*, 1983, *140*, 1058–1060.

Bolelli, G., Lafisca, S., Flamigni, C., Lodi, S., Franceschetti, F., Filicori, M., and Mosca, R. Heroin addiction: Relationship between the plasma levels of testosterone, dihydrotestosterone, androstenedione, LH, FSH, and the plasma concentration of heroin. *Toxicology*, 1979, *15*, 15–19.

Brady, J. P. and Bianco, F. C. Endorphins: Naloxone failure to increase sexual arousal in sexually unresponsive women: A Preliminary Report. *Biological Psychiatry*, 1980, *15*, 627–630.

Braude, M. C. and Morrison, J. M. *Preclinical toxicity studies of naltrexone. Narcotic Antagonists: Naltrexone. NIDA Research Monograph 9*. D. Julius and P. Renault (eds.), Rockville, Md., 1976.

Bruni, J. F., Van Vugt, D., Marshall, S., and Meites, J. Effects of naloxone, morphine, and methionine enkephalin on serum prolactin, luteinizing hormone, follicle-stimulating hormone, thyroid-stimulating hormone, and growth hormone. *Life Sciences*, 1977, *21*, 461–466.

Burroughs, W. S. *Junkie*. Ace, New York, 1953.

Chessick, R. D. The pharmacogenic orgasm in the drug addic. *Archives of General Psychiatry*, 1960, *3*, 117–128.

Cicero, T. J., Owens, D. P., Schomeker, P. F., and Meyer, E. R. Morphine-induced supersensitivity to the effects of naloxone on luteinizing hormone secretion in the male rat. *Journal of Pharmacology and Experimental Therapeutics*, 1983, *225*, 35–41.

Cicero, T. J., Meyer, R. R., and Schomeker, P. F. Development of tolerance to the effects of morphine on luteinizing hormone secretion as a function of castration in the male rat. *Journal of Pharmacology and Experimental Therapeutics*, 1982, *223*, 784–789.

Cicero, T. J., Meyer, E. R., Gabriel, S. M., and Wilcox, C. E. Androgenic-like effects of morphine in the male rat. *Proceedings of the 42nd Annual Scientific Meeting. Problems of Drug Dependence*, 1981, 152–158.

Cicero, T. J., Schainker, B. A., and Meyer, E. R. Endogenous opioids participate in the regulation of the hypothalamic-pituitary-luteinizing hormone axis and testosterone's feedback control of luteinizing hormone. *Endocrinology*, 1979, *104*, 1286–1291.

Cicero, T. J., Wilcox, C. E., Bell, R. D., and Meyer, E. R. Naloxone-induced increases in serum luteinizing hormone in the male: Mechanisms of action. *Journal of Pharmacology and Experimental Therapeutics*, 1979, *212*, 573–578.

Cicero, T. J. and Badger, T. M. A comparative analysis of the effects of narcotics, alcohol and the barbiturates on the hypothalamic-pituitary-gonadal axis. *Advances Experimental Medicine and Biology*, 1977, *85B*, 95–115.

Cicero, T. J., Badger, T. M., Wilcox, C. E., Bell, R. D., and Meyer, E. R. Morphine decreases luteinizing hormone by an action on the hypothalamic-pituitary axis. *Journal of Pharmacology and Experimental Therapeutics*, 1977a, *203*, 548–555.

Cicero, T. J., Bell, R. D., Meyer, E. R., and Schweitzer, J. Narcotics and the hypothalamic-pituitary-gonadal axis: Acute effects on luteinizing hormone, testosterone and androgen-dependent systems. *Journal of Pharmacology and Experimental Therapeutics*, 1977b, *201*, 76–83.

Cicero, T. J., Wilcox, C. E., Bell, R. D., and Meyer, E. R. Acute reductions in serum testosterone levels by narcotics in the male rat: Stereospecificity, blockade by naloxone and tolerance. *Journal of Pharmacology and Experimental Therapeutics*, 1976, *198*, 340–346.

Cicero, T. J., Meyer, E. R., Wiest, W. G., Olney, J. W., and Bell, R. D. Effects of chronic morphine administration on the reproductive system of the male rat. *Journal of Pharmacology and Experimental Therapeutics*, 1975, *192*, 542–548.

Cicero, T. J., Meyer, E. R., Bell, R. D., and Wiest, W. G. Effects of morphine on the secondary sex organs and plasma testosterone levels of rats. *Research Communications in Chemical Pathology and Pharmacology*, 1974, *7*, 17–24.

Cooper, A. J. and Ismail, A. A. A pilot study of mesterolone in impotence. *Psychopharmacology*, 1972, *26*, 379–386.

Craig, R. J. *Drug dependent patients*, 1973, *45*, 57–58, 173–196, 341, 356.

Crowley, T. J. and Simpson, R. Methadone dose and human sexual behavior. *International Journal of the Addictions*, 1978, *13*, 285–295.

Crowley, T. J., Hydinger, M., Stynes, A. J., and Feiger, A. Monkey motor stimulation and altered social behavior during chronic methadone adminstration. *Psychopharmacologia*, 1975, *43*, 135–144.

Crowley, T. J., Stynes, A. J., Hidinger, M., and Kaufman, I. C. Ethanol methamphetamine, pentobarbital, norephene, and monkey social behavior. *Archives of General Psychiatry*, 1974, *31*, 829–838.

Cushman, P. Plasma testosterone in narcotic addiction. *American Journal of Medicine*, 1973, *55*, 452–458.

Cushman, P. Sexual behavior in heroin addiction and methadone maintenance. *New York State Journal of Medicine*, 1972, 1261–1265.

DeLeon, G. and Wexler, H. K. Heroin addiction: Its relation to sexual behavior and sexual experience. *Journal of Abnormal Psychology*, 1973, *81*, 36–38.

Ellinwood, E. H., Smith, W. E., and Vaillant, G. E. *International Journal of the Addictions*, 1966, *1*, 44.

Espejo, R., Hogben, G., and Stimmel, B. Sexual performance of men on methadone maintenance. *Proceedings of 5th National Conference on Methadone Treatment*, 1973, *2*, 490–493.

Ferland, L., Fuxe, K., Eneroth, P., Gustafsson, J. A., and Skett, P. Effects of methionine-enkephalin on prolactin release and catecholamine levels and turnover in the median eminence. *European Journal of Pharmacology*, 1977, *43*, 89–90.

Fort, J. Heroin addiction among young men. *Psychiatry*, 1954, *17*, 251–259.

Garbutt, G., and Goldstein, A. Blind comparison of three methadone maintenance dosages in 180 patients. Proceedings of the 4th National Conference on Methadone Treatment. New York, 1972.

Gaulden, E. C., Littlefield, D. C., Putoff, O. E., and Seivert, A. L. Menstrual abnormalities associated with heroin addiction. *American Journal of Obstetrics and Gynecology,* 1964, *90,* 155–160.

Gay, G. R. and Sheppard, C. W. Sex-crazed dope fields—Myth or reality? *Drug Forum,* 1973, *2,* 125–140.

Gay, G. R., Newmeyer, J. A., Elion, R. A., and Wieder, S. The sensuous hippie part 1: Drug/sex practice in the Haight-Ashbury. *Drug Forum,* 1977, *6,* 27–47.

Gay, G. R., Newmeyer, J. A., Perry, M., Johnson, G., and Kurland, M. 1980–81. The sensuous hippie revisited: Drug/sex practices in San Francisco. *Journal of Psychoactive Drugs,* i982, *14,* 111–123.

Gessa, G. L. Induction of copulatory behavior in sexually inactive rats by naloxone. *Science,* 1979, *204,* 203–205.

Glick, B. B., Baughman, W. L., Jensen, J. N., and Pheonix, C. H. Endogenous opiate systems and primate reproduction. *Archives of Sexual Behavior,* 1982, *11,* 267–275.

Gold, M. S., Pottash, A. L. C., Extein, I., and Kleber, H. D. Dopamine and serum prolactin in methadone withdrawal. NIDA Research 34. Problems of Drug Dependence. Proceedings of the 42nd Annual Scientific Meeting, 1981, 367–372.

Gold, M. S., Redmond, D. E., and Donabedian, R. K. The effects of opiate agonist and antagonist on serum prolactin in primates: Possible role for endorphins in prolactin regulations. *Endocrinology,* 1979, *105,* 284–289.

Gold, M. S., Redmond, D. E., Donabedian, R. K., Goodwin, F. K., and Extein, I. Increase in serum prolactin by exogenous and endogenous opiates: Evidence for antidopamine and antipsychotic effects. *American Journal of Psychiatry,* 1978, *135,* 1415–1416.

Goldstein, A. and Hansteen, R. W. Evidence against involvement of endorphins in sexual arousal and orgasm in man. *Archives of General Psychiatry,* 1977, *34,* 1179–1180.

Grossman, A., Moult, P. J. A., McIntyre, H., Evans, J., Silverstone, T., Rees, L. H., and Besser, G. M. Opiate mediation of amenorrhea. *Clinical Endocrinology,* 1982, *17,* 379.

Guerra, F. Sex and drugs in the 16th Century. *British Journal of Addictions,* 1974, *69,* 269–289.

Hanbury, R., Cohen, M., and Stimmel, B. Adequacy of sexual performance in men maintained on methadone. *American Journal of Drug Alcohol Abuse,* 1977, *4,* 13–20.

Hudson, B. and Coghlan, J. P. Abnormalities of testosterone secretion in the male. In *Clinical Endocrinology,* E. B. Astwood and G. E. Cassidy (eds.), Grune and Stratton, New York, 1968, 562–568.

Hughes, H. *The Addict in the Street.* New York, Grove Press, 1967, 109.

Jackson, C. M. *The effects of inanition and malnutrition upon growth and structure.* P. Blakiston's Sons and Co., Philadelphia, 1925.

Kimura, Y., Miyata, K., Adachi, K., and Matsumura, S., The role of Alpha-andrenergic receptor mechanisms in ejaculation. *Tohoku Journal of Experimental Medicine,* 1972, *108,* 337–352.

LaBelle, F. S., Havlicek, V., Pinsky, C., and Leybin, L. Opiate-like, naloxone-reversible effects of androsterone sulfate in rats. *Canadian Journal of Physiology and Pharmacology*, 1978, 56, 940–944.

LaBelle, F. S. Opiate-specific displacement of steroid hormones from microsomes. *Life Sciences*, 1975, 16, 1783–1784.

Lafisca, S., Bolelli, G., Franceschetti, F., Filicori, M., Flamigni, C., and Marigo, M. Hormone levels in methadone-treated drug addicts. *Drug and Alcohol Dependence*, 1981, 8, 229–234.

Lal, H. B., Drawbaugh, R., Hynes, M., and Brown, G. Enhanced prolactin inhibition following chronic treatment with haloperidol and morphine. *Life Sciences*, 1977, 20, 101–106.

Litt, I. F. and Cohen, M. I. The drug-using adolescent as a pediatric patient. *The Journal of Pediatrics*, 1970, 77, 195–202.

Luttge, W. G. The role of gonadal hormones in the sexual behavior of the rhesus monkey and human. *Archives of Sexual Behavior*, 1971, 1, 61–85.

Malimnas, M. G. and Pomerantz, L. Pituitary replacement therapy in pseudo hypophysectomy. *Endocrinology*, 1941, 29, 558–562.

Mann, T. *The Biochemistry of Semen and of the Male Reproductive Tract*. J. Wiley and Sons, New York, 1964.

Marko, M. and Romer, D. Inhibitory effect of a new opioid agonist on reproductive endocrine activity in rats of both sexes. *Life Sciences* 1983, 33, 233–240.

Martin, C. A. and Martin, W. R. Opiate dependence in women. *Alcohol and Problems in Women*, New York, Plenum Publishing Co., 1980, 465–486.

Martin, W. R., Jasinski, D. R., Haertzen, C. A., Kay, D. C., Jones, B. E., Mansky, P. A., and Carpenter, R. W. Methadone—A reevaluation. *Archives of General Psychiatry*, 1973, 28, 286–295.

Mathis, J. L. Sexual aspects of heroin addiction. *Medical Aspects of Human Sexuality*, 1970, 4, 98–109.

McIntosh, T. K., Vallano, M. L., and Barfield, R. J. Effects of morphine, β-endorphin and naloxone on catecholamine levels and sexual behavior in the male rat. *Pharmacology Biochemistry & Behavior*, 1980, 13, 435–441.

Meites, J., Bruni, J. F. and Van Vugt, D. Effects of endogenous opiate peptides on release of anterior pituitary hormones. In: Collu, R., Barbeau, A., Ducharme, E. R., and Rochefort, G. G. (eds.). *Central Nervous System Effects of Hypothalamic Hormones and Other Peptides*. New York, Raven Press, 1979, 261–268.

Mendelson, J. H., Ellingboe, J., Kuehnle, J. C., and Mello, N. K. Effects of naltrexone on mood and neuroendocrine function in normal adult males. *Psychoneuroendocrinology*, 1979, 2, 231–236.

Mendelson, J. H., Ellingboe, J., Kuehnle, J. C., and Mello, N. K. Heroin and naltrexone effects on pituitary-gonadal hormones in man. *Journal of Pharmacology and Experimental Therapeutics*, 1980a, 214, 503–506.

Mendelson, J. H., Ellingboe, J., Kuehnle, J. C., and Mello, N. K. Heroin and naltrexone effects on pituitary-gonadal hormones in man: Tolerance and supersensitivity. Problems of Drug Dependence. *Proceedings of 41st Annual Scientific Meeting of the Committee on Durg Dependence*, 1980b NIDA Research Monograph Series #27.

Mendelson, J. H. and Mello, N. K. Plasma testosterone levels during chronic heroin use and protracted abstinence. *Clinical Pharmacology and Therapeutics*, 1975, *17*, 529–533.

Mendelson, J. H., Mendelson, J. E., and Patch, V. D. Plasma testosterone levels in heroin addiction and during methadone maintenance. *Journal of Pharmacology and Experimental Therapeutics*, 1975a, *192*, 211–217.

Mendelson, J. H., Meyer, R. E., Ellingboe, J., Mirin, S. M., and McDougle, M. Effects of heroin and methadone on plasma cortisol and testosterone. *Journal of Pharmacology and Experimental Therapeutics*, 1975b, *195*, 296–302.

Meyerson, B. J. and Terenius, L. Endorphin and male sexual behavior. *European Journal of Pharmacology*, 1977, *42*, 191–192.

Mirin, S. M., Mendelson, J. H., Ellingboe, J., and Meyer, R. E. Acute effects of heroin and naltrexone on testosterone and gonadotropin secretion: A pilot study. *Psychoneuroendocrinology*, 1976, *1*, 359–369.

Money, J. and Ehrhardt, A. A. *Man and women, boy and girl.* The differention and dimorphism of gender identity from conception to maturity, John Hopkins Press, Baltimore, 1973.

Mulinas, M. G. and Pomerantz, L. Pituitary replacement therapy in pseudohypophysectomy. *Endocrinology*, 1941, *29*, 558–562.

Muraki, T., Nakadate, H., Tokunaga, Y., Kato, R., and Makino, T. Effect of narcotic analgesics and naloxone on proestrous surges of LH, FSH, and Prolactin in rats. *Neuroendocrinology*, 1979, *28*, 241–247.

Muraki, T., Tokunaga, Y., and Makino, T. Effects of morphine and naloxone on serum LH, FSH and prolactin levels and on hypothalamic content of LH-RF in proestrous rats. *Endocrinology Japan*, 1977, *24*, 313–315.

Murphy, M. R. Evidence for the involvement of endogenous opiates in male sexual behavior. *Sexology: Sexual Biology, Behavior and Therapy.* Selected papers of the 5th World Congress of Sexology, Jerusalem, Israel, 1981a, 53–57.

Murphy, M. R. Methadone reduces sexual performance and sexual motivation in the male Syrian golden hamster. *Pharmacology Biochemistry & Behavior*, 1981b, *14*, 561–567.

Myers, B. M. and Baum, M. J. Facilitation by opiate antagonists of sexual performance in the male rat. *Pharmacology Biochemistry & Behavior*, 1979, *10*, 615–618.

Pace, J. L. and Podesta, M. T. The Anatomical distribution of diverticula of the large intestine based on post-morten studies. *Anatomical Record*, 1974, *178*, 434–435.

Packman, P. M. and Rothchild, J. A. Morphine inhibition of ovulation: Reversal by naloxone. *Endocrinology*, 1976, *99*, 7–10.

Palmer, M. R., Seiger, A., Hoffer, B. J., and Olson, L. Modulatory interactions between enkephalin and catecholamines: Anatomical and physiological substrates. *Federation Proceedings*, 1983, *42*, 2934–2946.

Pang, C. N., Zimmerman, E., and Sawyer, C. H. Effects of morphine on the proestrous surge of luteinizing hormone in the rat. *Anatomical Record*, 1974, *178*, 434.

Parr, D. Sexual aspects of drug abuse in narcotic addicts. *British Journal of Addiction*, 1975, *71*, 261–268.

Pelligrini Quarantotti, B. P., Corda, M. G., Paglietti, E., Biggio, G., and Gessa, G. L. Inhibition of copulatory behavior in male rats by d-Ala-met-enkephalinamide. *Life Sciences*, 1978, *23*, 673–678.

Perlmutter, J. F. Maternal morbidity in the pregnant drug addict. In *Drug abuse in pregnancy and neonatal effects,* Joseph L. Rementeria, (ed.), 1977, St. Louis, The C.V. Mosby Company.

Rado, S. The psychic effects of intoxicants: An attempt to evolve a psychoanalytical theory of morbid cravings. *International Journal of Psychoanalysis,* 1926, *7,* 396–413.

Reid, R. L., Hoff, J. D., Yen, S. S. C., and Li, C. H. Effects of exogenous β-endorphin on pituitary hormone secretion and its disappearance rate in normal human subjects. *Journal of Clinical Endocrinology and Metabolism,* 1981, *52,* 1179–1184.

Rotsztejn, W. H., Drouva, S. V., Pattou, E., and Kordan, C. Effects of morphine on the basal and the dopamine-induced release of LHRH from mediobasal hypothalamic fragments in vitro. *Journal of Pharmacology,* 1978, *50,* 285–286.

Rotsztejn, W. H., Drova, S. V., Pattou, E., and Kordan, C. Metenkephalin inhibits in vitro dopamine-induced LHRH release from mediobasal hypothalamus of male rats. *Nature,* 1978, *274,* 281–283.

Sachs, B. D., Valcourt, R. J., and Flagg, H. C. Copulatory behavior and sexual reflexes of male rats treated with naloxone. *Pharmacology Biochemistry & Behavior,* 1980, *14,* 251–253.

Santen, R. J., Sofsky, J., Bilic, N., and Lippert, R. Mechanism of action of narcotics in the production of menstrual dysfunction in women. *Fertility and Sterility,* 1975, *26,* 538–548.

Schiavi, R. C. and White, D. Androgens and male sexual function: A review of human studies. *Journal Sex Marital Therapy,* 1976, *2,* 214–228.

Shaar, C. G., Frederickson, R. C., Dininger, N. B., and Jackson, L. Enkephalin analogues and naloxone modulate the release of growth hormone and prolactin evidence for regulation by an endogenous opioid peptide in brain. *Life Sciences,* 1977, *21,* 853.

Smith, D. E., Moser, C., Wesson, D. R., Apter, M., Buxton, M. E., Davison, J. V., Orgel, M., and Buffum, J. A clinical guide to the diagnosis and treatment of heroin-related sexual dysfunction. *Journal of Psychoactive Drugs,* 1982, *14,* 91–99.

Snyder, S. H. Opiate receptor in normal and drug altered brain function. *Nature,* 1975, *257,* 185–189.

Stoffer, S. S. A gynecologic study of drug addicts. *American Journal of Gynecology,* 1968, *101,* 779–783.

Sylvester, P. W., Chen, H. T., and Meites, J. Effects of morphine and naloxone on phasic release of luteinizing hormone and follicle-stimulating hormone. *Proceedings of the Society for Experimental Biology and Medicine,* 1980, *164,* 207–211.

Tagliamonte, A., Fratta, W., DelFiacco, M., and Gessa, G. L. Possible stimulatory role of brain dopamine in the copulatory behavior of male rats. Brief Communication. *Pharmacology Biochemistry & Behavior,* 1973, *2,* 257–260.

TenHouten, S. Sexual Dynamics and strength of heroin addiction. *Journal of Psychoactive Drugs,* 1982, *14,* 101–109.

Terry, C. E. and Pellens, M. *The Opium Problem,* 1928. repr. Paterson Smith, Montclair, New Jersey, 1970.

Thomas, J. A. and Dombrosky, J. T. Effects of methadone on the male reproduction system. *Archives Internationales de Pharmacodynamie et de Therapie*, 1975, *215*, 215–221.

Tokunaga, Y., Muraki, T., and Hosoya, E. Effects of repeated morphine administration on copulation and on the hypothalamic-pituitary gonadal axis of male rats. *Japanese Journal of Pharmacology*, 1977, *27*, 65–70.

Tolis, G., Hickey, J. and Guyda, H. Effects of morphine on serum growth hormone, cortisol, prolactin, and thyroid stimulating hormone in man. *Clinical Endocrinology and Metabolism*, 1975, *41*, 797–800.

Vrbicky, K. W., Baumstark, J. S., Wells, I. C., Hilgers, T. W., Kable, W. T., and Elias, C. J. Evidence of the involvement of β-endorphin in the human menstrual cycle. *Fertility and Sterility*, 1982, *38*, 701–704.

Wallach, R. C., Jerez, E., and Glinick, G. Pregnancy and menstrual function in narcotics addicts treated with methadone. *American Journal of Obstetrics and Gynecology*, 1969, *105*, 1226–1229.

Wieland, W. F. and Yunger, M. Sexual effects and side effects of heroin and methadone. Department of Health, Education, and Welfare, *Public Health Service Publication 2172*, 1971.

Wilkes, M. M. and Yen, S. S. C. Augmentation by naloxone of efflux of LRF from superfused medical basal hypothalamus. *Life Sciences*, 1981, *28*, 2355–2359.

Wikler, A. and Rasor, M. M. Psychiatric aspects of drug addiction. *American Journal of Medicine*, 1953, *14*, 566–570.

Young, W. C. *Sex and Internal Secretions*. Krieger, Huntington N.Y., 1973.

Zubiran, S. and Gomez-Mont, F. Endocrine disturbances in chronic malnutrition. *Vitamins and Hormones*, 1953, *11*, 97–132.

Chapter 14

Tobacco

Tobacco is one of the most widely used substances in the world. The main ingredient in tobacco responsible for its use is nicotine, a colorless to pale yellow liquid which is very soluble in water and lipids. Nicotine has a low boiling point and therefore vaporizes quickly as tobacco burns.

Nicotine is rapidly absorbed from the lungs after inhalation. About 10 percent of the nicotine present in a cigarette is actually absorbed with the result that only about 0.2 mg is taken into the body per cigarette. After absorption, nicotine is rapidly distributed to all tissues.

The main psychological effect of nicotine is stimulation of the brain although smokers often feel relaxed. Heart rate is increased and blood pressure is increased whereas blood flow to the extremities is decreased.

The mechanism of nicotine's action in the peripheral nervous system involves an initial stimulation of neuronal activity followed by a blockade due to depolarization of nerve fibers. This results in a relaxation of skeletal muscles and may be responsible in part for the sense of overall relaxation associated with smoking. In addition to mimicking the effects of acetylcholine, nicotine also causes the adrenal gland to release epinephine which in turn results in various effects associated with adenergic stimulation, e.g., constriction of blood vessels.

MALE SEXUALITY

Soon after its introduction to Europeans in the sixteenth century, tobacco became the center of controversy concerning its effects on libido, generative function, and offspring of those who smoked. In some instances, such as in the Turkish Empire, feelings ran to such extremes that in 1622 the Sultan, Murad IV, made smoking a crime punishable by death! The reason for this draconian measure was the Sultan's belief that smoking made people infertile (Maynwaring, 1669).

Anecdotal Reports

The first written pronouncement that smoking tobacco could result in sterility occurred in 1601 in a book entitled *Work for Chimny-Sweepers*. Its author, an anonymous writer whose pen name was Philaretes, was opposed to smoking in general and specifically took aim at smoking's effects on reproductive function:

> . for certaine proofe that Tobacco dryeth up the sperme & seed of man, I heare by faithfull relation of such as have much used it; That wereas before the use thereof, they had bene long molested with a fluxe of seed . . . they were in short space eased of this affect by the onely use of this medicine. For no doubt, this fierie fume, dried up the superfluitie of that matter. . . .
>
> (Philaretes, 1936)

One of the reasons Philaretes and many others believed that smoking was so harmful was because tobacco smoke was so hot and dry that it vaporized the vital fluids of the body.

About a quarter of a century later, in 1626, William Vaughan concluded his own revised treatise on the medical properties of tobacco with a rhyme he hoped would help his readers refrain from smoking:

Tobacco, that outlandish weede,
It spends the braine, and spoiles the seede:
It duls the spirite, it dims the sight,
It robs a woman of her right.

(Quoted by Brooks, 1937)

But other authors disagreed, contending that there was no proof whatsoever for such accusations. Using a similar poetic format Barclay wrote several years earlier that there was no substance to such beliefs:

Some do this plant with odious crymes disgrace,
And call the poore Tabacco homicid,
They say that it, O what a monstrous cace!
Forestals the life, and kils man in the seed,
....
Good Ladie looke not to these raving speiches,
You know by proof that all these blames are lies,
Forged by scurvie leud unlearned Leiches
As time hath taught, and practise that all tryes.
Tobacco neither altereth health nor hew,
Ten thousand thousands know that it is true.

(Quoted by Brooks, 1937)

In Holland, Dr. Cornelius Bontekoe attempted to reconcile both of these positions. Writing in 1685, he pointed out that the reason many smokers may be sterile is that they do not eat well or they engage in physical excesses (Brooks, 1937).

Next to sterility, many authors claimed that smoking tobacco dampened the libido. A few writers, however, were of the opposite opinion. In his history of the new colony of Virginia (1615), Hamor alluded to the possible aphrodisiac effects of the plant: "We observe that those Indians which have one, two, or more women, take much [tobacco]—but such as yet have no appropriate woman take little or none at all" (Hamor, 1849).

In 1633, Swedish author Jacob Olaf Hernodius recommended tobacco outright as an aphrodisiac for "those cold and inept in the cause of love" (quoted by Brooks, 1937). But most other writers considered tobacco an anaphrodisiac. In 1690, an anonymous compiler of anecdotes cited a woman who attributed her husband's reduced sexual ardor to his use of tobacco. In 1722, in *Venus Rebutted*, the same observation was independently made (Brooks, 1937). In Italy, in 1758, author Casimiro Affaitati specifically recommended tobacco as an anaphrodisiac, especially to those wishing to live in celibacy, because it "decayed the generative powers" (quoted by Brooks, 1937). During the hearings on the canonization of Saint Joseph of Cupertino, one of the minor objections brought forward was that Saint Joseph used tobacco for just this reason: "The assiduous use of tobacco restrains lust as I myself have heard concerning Father Joseph of Cupertino. . . . He uses tobacco not only to keep awake at night for vigils, but also to resist the temptation of the flesh and to overcome the danger of yielding to human frailty" (quoted by Brooks, 1937). In 1669, Benedetto Stella wrote that churchmen should use tobacco because of its effects on the libido and cited Saint Joseph as an example:

> . . . the use of tobacco taken in moderation is not only useful but even necessary for preachers, monks, brothers, and other religious who ought and desire to lead a chaste life and repress sensual emotions. Because the natural cause of libidinousness is heat and dampness, and since, with the use of tobacco this cause is dried up, the users do not feel these libidinous emotions so vehemently. Tobacco, therefore, should not be used by married people. For these reasons take tobacco in imitation of the great Servant of God of our times, Father Joseph da Cupertino. . . (Quoted by Brooks, 1937)

In more recent writings on the subject, tobacco has been also credited more with dampening than arousing the libido. In 1849, an American author of sex manuals stated that tobacco caused impotence (Hollick, 1850). In 1933, Schrottenback coined the term "nicotine impotence" for the loss of libido allegedly due to smoking (Sterling & Kobayashi, 1975). Clinical case studies form the early 1900s also cited evidence that diminished libido was reversed once abstinence occurred. Whereas most of these latter case studies were in agreement about smoking's effects on male sexuality, none seems to have been based on any data that would be acceptable by present-day standards. In terms of smoking and female sexuality, there is virtually no information available, anecdotal or otherwise. A number of studies have begun to appear concerning tobacco's effects on reproductive function and a few preliminary survey studies have been reported concerning smoking and sexual activity. Most of the research efforts have concerned tobacco's or nicotine's affects on hormones and ovulation in animals.

Clinical Studies

There are few clinical or epidemiological reports of the relation between smoking and sex. Ochsner (1977) cited three cases in which he claimed an increase in libido followed abstinence from smoking. A similar increase in libido was noted by Subak-Sharpe (1974) in a patient who gave up smoking.

Two retrospective studies have noted decreased sexual function associated with smoking. In France, Cendron and Vallery-Masson (1970) compared the sexual activity of 70 men, aged 45–90. The men were divided into two groups on the basis of whether they smoked at 25 and 40 years of age. Self-reported sexual activity was lower among smokers than nonsmokers at the two ages. Although the authors indicated that this relationship could have been due to many factors, they contended that it was not inconceivable that smoking may have a depressant effect on libido.

In Czechoslovakia, Mellan (1963) studied patients from the Sexualogical Institute of the Charles University in Prague and found a greater number of "heavy" smokers were "sexually defective," e.g., fear of intercourse, premature ejaculation, compared to nonsmokers and light smokers. However, the two groups differed on several parameters, including age, and Mellan felt that there was not enough evidence to conclude unequivocally that smoking was a causal factor in producing "sexual defects."

Some studies suggest that sexual experience occurs at an earlier age among smokers. In Czechoslovakia, Raboch and Mellan noted that sexual experience among males and females 15–19 years of age was more common among smokers than nonsmokers.

In a brief study of American adolescents aged 14 to 17 years of age, Malcolm and Shephard (1978) found male smokers engaged in sexual intercourse more frequently, had more sexual partners, and had more liberal attitudes toward sex than male nonsmokers. A similar trend was noted for female smokers (see Table 17).

One reason for the greater sexual activity among adolescents who smoke may be an earlier onset of puberty as reported by Lall and co-workers (1980). In a study of 1000 schoolboys aged 8–16 in India, Lall determined that puberty occurred about a half-year earlier in smokers. However, secondary sex characteristics, e.g., pubic, axillary, and facial hair, appeared at a significantly later age among smokers.

"Masculinity" (defined in terms of external morphological features) was reported as being less characteristic of smokers than nonsmokers by Seltzer (1959). The relationship between masculinity ratings and smoking was dose-related. Only 3.3 percent of the nonsmokers in this study had some degree of "weakness" of masculine component compared to 9.6 percent for moderate smokers and 17.2 percent for heavy smokers.

The only clinical study relating the effects of smoking and sexual function is that of Forsberg and his co-workers (1979). In this brief report two men, aged 20 and 27, who consulted a clinic because of erectile dysfunction, were advised to stop smoking. After abstaining from smoking for a few days, erectile capacity was

TABLE 17.   Sexual Attitudes and Behavior of Adolescent (14–17 years old) Smokers and Nonsmokers (%)[a]

Group	Premarital sex is immoral	Frequency of intercourse			Number of sex partners			
		0	1–2	2	0	1	2–5	6
Male smokers (N = 24)	29.2	13.6	50.0	36.4	8.7	34.8	26.1	35.8
Male nonsmokers (N = 34)	30.3	84.8	6.1	9.1	84.8	12.1	0.0	3.0
Female smokers (N = 27)	25.9	59.3	11.1	29.6	63.0	18.5	0.0	
Female nonsmokers (N = 50)	53.3	65.3	16.3	18.3	65.3	20.4	10.2	4.1

[a]Data from Malcolm and Shephard (1978).

restored. Blood pressure measurements, determined prior to and after cessation of smoking, indicated that systolic penile blood pressure was increased after smoking abstinence. The authors proposed that smoking caused erectile impotence by causing vasoconstriction in the penile vasculature and that there is individual vulnerability to this effect, which accounts for the impairment of erection only in a small proportion of male smokers.

Studies in Animals

There are a number of studies in which male animals injected with nicotine display behavior toward females that supports the overall impression from the human literature of an overall decrease in sexual activity associated with tobacco and its ingredients.

The one exception is the study reported by Soulairac and Soulairac (1972). Soulairac injected male rats with nicotine (0.6 or 1.2 mg/kg, s.c.) and observed their behavior toward females 30 minutes later. Animals injected with the higher dose did not engage in sexual behavior and appeared to experience mild convulsive effects. Animals injected with the lower dose exhibited increased sexual activity over "normal" levels, e.g., increased number of ejaculations, decreased ejaculatory latency, decreased refractory period between mountings, decreased latency to mount. Nicotine was also reported to increase vigor of pelvic thrusting and increased the precision of intromissions so that nicotine-injected animals had fewer "false intromissions." The duration of the effect was approximately two hours. The authors related this effect to nicotine's stimulation of cholinergic mechanisms underlying sexual behavior in the rat.

However, the unequivocal assessment of these results in the Soulairac study is precluded because of numerous methodological flaws, among which were the failure to inject animals in the nontreated condition with vehicle, and the failure to test males with females known to be sexually receptive. Testing animals in the drug condition after previously testing them in a nondrug condition also confounds a "practice" effect with drug treatment.

A more methodologically rigorous study of nicotine's effects on male sexual behavior in the rat was reported by Bignami (1966). In this study, females were brought into estrus with estradiol and progesterone, and female sexual receptivity was verified by pre-testing with males other than those given nicotine. Experimental males were previously given sexual experience with other females. Testing began 20 minutes after subcutaneous injection of nicotine tartrate (0.1, 0.2, 0.5, 1.0, or 2.0 mg/kg).

Doses of 0.1 or 0.2 mg/kg did not affect sexual contact latency, intromission latency, mount frequency, intromissions, latency between intromissions, or postejaculatory refractory period. Doses of 0.5, 1.0, and 2.0 mg/kg decreased several indices of sexual behavior (intromission latency, intromission frequency, and postejaculatory refractory interval) but did not affect other indices. This effect may have been due to depression of motor activity and general malaise, although the authors indicate that most animals mated following injection.

Cattanach (1962) reported that subcutaneous injection of nicotine (6.7 mg/kg) for six weeks prior to mating did not affect the number of matings in mice. Male fertility was also not affected as indicated by litter size, implantation sites, or pre-implantation losses.

EFFECTS ON SPERM

Human Studies

Few studies have reported abnormal sperm samples associated with tobacco usage. Sperm counts have been reported to be lowered as a result of smoking in some studies, but not in others. Decreased sperm motility, however, has been reported in several studies as a result of smoking. In an early case report, Phillips (1943) reported that the sperm count of a 33-year-old male who smoked 20 to 30 cigarettes a day was normal but the man's sperm lacked any motility. After the patient gave up smoking for a month, sperm motility increased and his wife became pregnant. When he resumed smoking again, sperm motility again ceased. Abstinence from smoking once again resulted in normal sperm motility.

Schirren (1972) reported that sperm count was not affected by smoking in a group of men (N = 4372) with sexual dysfunction. After a subgroup (N=10) of patients abstained from smoking for 2 to 6 months, their sperm motility increased considerably.

Viczian (1968) reported that sperm motility was lower in smokers compared to nonsmokers and the extent of the decrease in motility was dose related: men smoking 30 or more cigarettes per day had a sperm motility of 49 percent compared to 57 percent for men who smoked 10 cigarettes or less per day. Sperm motility for nonsmokers was 69 percent.

Reduced sperm motility and sperm density among smokers compared to nonsmokers were also noted by Campbell and Harrison (1979) in their study of 253 men attending an infertility clinic.

Evans and his co-workers (1981) compared sperm samples from 43 smokers with those from 43 nonsmokers. Subjects all attended an infertility clinic and patients were excluded if there was a history of other factors associated with sperm abnormality, e.g., alcoholism; exposure to toxic chemicals or radiation; undescended testicles at any age; variocele, hormone, or drug treatment. Smokers had a significantly higher proportion of abnormal sperm than nonsmokers (46% versus 42%, respectively) and also lower sperm counts. Among the observed abnormalities were very large or very small sperm, sperm with multiple heads or tails, and immature sperm.

In contrast to the Evans report, Godfrey (1981) was unable to detect any relationship between smoking and proportion of abnormal sperm among men attending an infertility clinic in a study of 344 men.

These data suggest that smoking may be an important factor in reducing sperm motility for some men but that there is no conclusive evidence that smoking produces abnormal sperm. Data from animal studies also fail to support the latter possibility (Cattanach, 1962). As suggested by Schirren (1970) and Forsberg *et al.* (1979), there may be an individual sensitivity to tobacco products evident when sperm samples from individual men are studied, even though samples from smokers and nonsmokers may not differ statistically. This possibility is especially interesting in light of case reports in which abstinence from smoking resulted in increases in sperm motility and sperm count.

Studies in Animals

Early studies of tobacco's and nicotine's effects on spermatogenesis in animals are reviewed by Larson (1961). In general, these studies seem to document a deleterious effect of these agents on spermatogenesis and sperm activity, but, in most cases, there were no control procedures for tobacco- or nicotine-related undernutrition so drug activity was confounded with inanition. There were also some inconsistencies between these studies. Stadtlander (1936), for instance, was unable to observe any effects of a twice daily subcutaneous injection regimen of nicotine pierate (0.1 mg) in mice treated for several months. Wilson and his co-workers (1937) reported that 12 out of 22 rats ingesting diets containing nicotine tannate and only 1 rat out of 23 ingesting nicotine bentonite were aspermic, while 3 out of 5 control rats placed on food restriction were aspermic. In contrast to these results, Erbacher & coworkers (1940) noted aspermia in rats subcutaneously injected daily with nicotine (0.05 mg) for 20 to 40 days. This dose was sufficient to cause convulsions. Decreased spermatogenesis was observed by day 20 of treatment. Animals receiving lower doses of 0.025 or 0.005 mg did not exhibit observable changes in spermatogenesis.

More recent studies in animals have reported adverse effects on sperm production but again there has been a confounding between drug administration and food intake. In addition, another source of confounding has been noted in conjunction with the test procedures used to expose animals to tobacco smoke.

Viczian (1968) placed mature male rats in a smoking chamber for 15 minutes, 8 times daily, for 6 weeks. At the end of the 6-week exposure period, animals were sacrificed and compared with non-treated males. Animals exposed to cigarette smoke lost about 10–15 grams in body weight and had more immature sperms (more primary spermatocytes and more abnormal mitotic spermatocytes) than control rats. The number of old spermatocytes was also increased, whereas number of spermatids was reduced. Nuclear volume of spermatids was also reduced. These data were interpreted as indicating inhibition of spermatogenesis through interference with mitosis in spermatocytes. However, it is not clear whether these results occurred directly as a result of tobacco smoke exposure, or indirectly through loss of body weight associated with exposure to smoke.

Sperm motility was inhibited by nicotine in a dose-related manner in sea urchins. Concentrations of 0.15 to 0.25 percent reduced and ultimately inhibited motility to the point that sperm were no longer able to fertilize ova (Longo and Anderson, 1970).

In some instances, the results of these studies may be due to an artifact as indicated by a study reported by Dontewill and co-workers (1973). An important confounding in most studies involving exposure to cigarette smoke on reproductive function is that control animals are untreated, i.e., they are not placed in the same apparatus as experimental animals. When male hamsters were exposed to cigarette smoke five times a week for up to 100 weeks, Dontewill and co-workers were unable to observe any effects of exposure *per se* on testes weights or testicular atrophy. However, restraining animals in the holding tube did result in a decrease in testicular weight.

Decreases in testicular weights following treatment with tobacco or nicotine were reported in several early studies (see review by Larson *et al.*, 1961). However, in most instances, there were no controls for decreased food intake or restraint. Doses were also very large and changes also occurred in other organs, so that in general these results were probably the indirect result of general malaise rather than the direct effect of these substances. In addition to Dontewill's (1973) report indicating decreased testicular weight resulting from restraint, Wilson and co-workers (1937) noted that similar changes to those resulting from exposure to nicotine resulted when animals were food-deprived. In their review of the literature in this area, Larson and his co-workers (1961) likewise agree that many of the degenerative changes observed in animals treated with nicotine were the result of "general trophic disturbances."

There have been no recent studies of nicotine's effects on penile function in animals. Early studies in this area are reviewed by Larson *et al.* (1961). In general, these early studies suggest that nicotine may have an inhibitory effect on penile excitability. Henderson and Roepke (cited by Larson) reported that intravenous injection of 10 mg of nicotine inhibited dilation in the dog penis, which ordinarily occurs following stimulation of the nerve fibers passing in the peritoneum from the rectum to the prostate. In another study by Tournade and co-workers (cited by Larson *et al.*), electrical stimulation of the erector nerve in dogs that inhaled cigarette smoke resulted in only partial erection, although effects on bladder and rectum were undiminished.

In summary, studies in animals indicate that exposure to tobacco smoke and nicotine can result in adverse effects on spermatogenesis, but these effects appear to be the indirect result of such exposure. The same is true of previously reported effects on the testes. The reported effects on erector function, however, are less likely to be indirectly mediated and warrant further investigation since they may provide additional information concerning similar loss of function in human smokers (see above).

Effects on Hormones

Effects on Androgens

Surprisingly, there have been very few studies of the effects of smoking on male sex hormones. Briggs (1973) compared a small group (N=6) of smokers (30 cigarettes per day or more) and nonsmokers (N=6) matched for age, height, weight, marital status, and occupation. Plasma testosterone levels were significantly lower in the smokers. One week after abstaining from smoking, plasma testosterone levels in smokers increased significantly. In a brief study of the relation between smoking and testosterone levels, Perksy and his co-workers (1977) observed a negative correlation between amount of cigarettes smoked and reduction in testosterone levels. In contrast to these observations, Winternitz and Quillen (1977) did not observe any acute effects of smoking on blood testosterone levels in male smokers. In this study, blood testosterone levels were assessed prior to smoking, during smoking, and after smoking. There were also no significant changes associated with smoking in luteinizing hormone or in follicle stimulating hormone levels in these men.

No effects of nicotine (2 mg/kg, 4 times) on basal serum levels of luteinizing hormone and prolactin in male rats were noted by Fuxe and his co-workers (1977).

FEMALE SEXUALITY

In contrast to the many anecdotes and early clinical warnings concerning the effects of smoking on male libido and sexual function, there is nothing similar in the way of smoking and female libido. In recent years, however, numerous studies have been conducted exploring the effects of exposure to cigarette smoke or nicotine on reproductive function and physiology. Prior to surveying this body of information, a study of nicotine's actions on sexual behavior in the female rat warrants some attention because it is the only one of its kind, and because of its findings.

Ovariectomized rats were initially treated with estradiol for 5 days, following which they were intraperitoneally injected with nicotine (0.01, 0.05, 0.10, or 0.25 mg/kg). Sexual behavior was not affected by the lowest dose. The 0.10 mg/kg dose increased sexual "soliciting" (hopping, darting, earwiggling) and lordosis the most. Lordosis was also increased by the 0.25 mg/kg dose, but this increase was attributed to depression of motor activity resulting in passive acceptance of the male. Mecamylamine, a cholinergic antagonist, antagonized the increase in sexual responsiveness if administered shortly before nicotine. The authors interpreted these data as evidence that nicotine acted as a replacement for progesterone (since estrogen plus progesterone induces sexual behavior in the female rat), or that nicotine increased sensitivity to estrogen (Fuxe *et al.*, 1977).

Some of the earliest studies of tobacco's effects on reproduction investigated potential changes in ovaries in animals (Larson *et al.*, 1961). In many instances, ovarian degeneration, as well as degeneration and destruction of mature follicles, were observed. Other studies reported that high doses of nicotine, e.g., 12–15 mg/kg, reduced or eliminated reproductive cycles in animals, whereas lower doses were without effect. Subsequent studies indicated that the changes in reproductive function produced by nicotine were probably the result of nicotine-related decreases in food intake resulting in undernutrition.

EFFECTS ON HORMONES

More recent studies (summarized in Table 18) have indicated that nicotine may affect reproductive function via hormonal mechanisms.

Blake and his co-workers have conducted several studies of nicotine's effects on various hormones involved in reproductive function. In one study, nicotine (2 mg) was injected subcutaneously in rats on the day of proestrus. The normal proestrus surge of luteinizing hormone was delayed by 90 minutes and peak levels of the hormone were lowered and of shorter duration compared to controls. Ovulation was not inhibited, however (Blake *et al.*, 1972a). In another study, administration of 5 mg/kg over a period of 7 hours did inhibit ovulation (Blake *et al.*, 1972b).

McLean and his co-workers (1977) have likewise demonstrated that tobacco smoke is capable of affecting the release of luteinizing hormone from the pituitary. In this study, adult female rats were initially cannulated and were then exposed to cigarette smoke from

TABLE 18. Effects of Nicotine and Cigarette Smoke on Luteinizing Hormone Release in Female Rats

Source	Dosage	Effect	Comment
Blake *et al.* (1972a)	2 mg per rat, s.c.	↓	Delayed release during proestrus, decreased peak levels
Blake (1974)		—	No effect in conjunction with luteinizing hormone-releasing hormone
Eneroth *et al.* (1977)	2 mg, 4 times, i.p.	↓	Delayed release in animals treated with pregnant mare serum gonadotropin
McClean *et al.* (1977)	Cigarette smoke	↓	Delay in peak levels during proestrus

cigarettes containing a high (2.5 mg nicotine/cigarette) or low (0.32 mg nicotine/cigarette) nicotine content. Exposure occurred in a smoking chamber for three 15-minute periods separated by rest periods of 15 minutes. Animals were exposed on the morning of proestrus. A total of 11.25 or 1.44 mg nicotine was delivered to the smoking chamber in the two conditions respectively, with 6 to 8 animals being exposed at the same time. Control animals were subjected to the same chamber and handling procedures except for smoke inhalation. Exposure to the higher nicotine condition delayed the surge of luteinizing hormone as compared to controls. Exposure to the low dose had minimal effects.

Blake and co-workers (1974) injected female rats with luteinizing hormone-releasing hormone in addition to nicotine. Under these conditions luteinizing hormone levels were not affected, indicating that the site of nicotine's inhibitory effect on release of luteinizing hormone is probably in the hypothalamus.

As a result of their studies, Eneroth and co-workers (1977) hypothesize that nicotine's inhibitory effects on luteinizing hormone is related to an increase in dopamine turnover in the area of the hypothalamus where luteinizing hormone-releasing hormone is concentrated and that the activity of this dopaminergic system is under control of nicotine-mediated cholinergic receptors.

Since luteinizing hormone affects ovulation, inhibition with its release ought to be paralleled by an inhibitory effect on ovulation. Although Blake and co-workers (1972a) were unable to detect any significant effects of nicotine on ovulation, such an effect was observed in rats exposed to tobacco smoke by McLean and his co-workers (1977).

Luteinizing hormone, however, is primarily responsible for causing the release of ova from the ovary. Failure to observe effects of nicotine when administration is given at time of proestrus might only have a delaying effect on ovulation. In this regard, Eneroth and co-workers did not observe any significant changes in follicle stimulating hormones levels in ovariectomized rats or in female rats treated with pregnant mare serum gonadotropin (Eneroth *et al.*, 1977).

TABLE 19.   Effects of Cigarette Smoke and Nicotine on Prolactin in Female Rats

Source	Dosage	Effect	Comments
Blake *et al.* (1971c)	1 mg twice, s.c.	↓	Suckling-induced release
Blake *et al.* (1972a)	1 mg/kg, twice, s.c.	↓	Delayed release during proestrus, basal levels were depressed
Eneroth *et al.* (1977)	2 mg/kg, 4 times, s.c.	↓	Decrease in hypersecretion induced by pregnant mare serum gonadotropin
Eneroth *et al.* (1977)	2 mg/kg, 4 times, i.p.	—	Basal levels unaffected
		↓	Reduction in increase produced by α-methyl tyrosine
Ferry *et al.* (1974)	Cigarette smoke	↓	Delay in suckling-induced release during proestrus
McClean *et al.* (1977)	Cigarette smoke	—	No effect on timing or peak levels

Prolactin

In most studies (summarized in Table 19) nicotine has been found to reduce secretion of prolactin in response to specific stimuli, e.g, nursing, pregnant mare serum gonadotropin. Basal levels were not affected in one study (Eneroth *et al.*, 1977), however, and in another cigarette smoke did not affect timing or amount of secretion during proestrus (McLean *et al.*, 1977).

In conjunction with nicotine's effects on prolactin secretion, Blake *et al.* (1972c) suggested that nicotine probably did not block milk secretion since milk could be observed in rat pups' stomachs at 10–60 minutes after nursing on nicotine-treated mothers. However, Ferry and his co-workers (1974) noted that, despite the presence of "milkspots" in the stomachs of such animals, pups from mothers exposed to cigarette smoke weighed less than control pups when weights were recorded prior to and after suckling.

FERTILITY

Higher infertility rates among women who smoke have been reported in several studies (Hammond, 1961; Pettersson *et al.*, 1973; Tokuhata, 1968; Vessey *et al.*, 1978). Tokuhata (1968) examined the smoking histories of 2,016 women and found 46 percent more instances of infertility among smokers than would be expected by chance after adjustment for factors such as husband's smoking habits, cause of death, e.g., cancer, marriage. Among women who smoked and whose husbands did not smoke, there was a 23 percent infertility rate. Among women who did not smoke and whose husbands did smoke, the infertility rate was 13 percent.

The means by which smoking may be affecting fertility in women has begun to be examined in animals. Neri and Marcus (1972) examined the effects of nicotine on fallopian tube activity in monkeys during the latter half of the menstrual cycle. Changes in such activity could affect the entry, migration, fertilization, or transfer of the ovum/conceptus to the uterus and therefore could be a factor in smoking-related infertility. Although intravenous injection of nicotine did not affect tubal tonus or amplitude of contraction, the frequency of burst was increased. Since the latter could affect the time for a fertilized ovum to reach the uterus, the authors propose that nicotine could act in this way to prevent implantation and thereby adversely affect fertility.

Card and Mitchell (1979) reported that subcutaneous administration of nicotine (5 mg/kg, twice daily) delayed implantation of the rat blastocyst in the uterus by about 9 hours. This effect was not due to delayed entrance of fertilized ova into the uterine lumen but could have been the result of decreased uterine receptivity. The number of blastocysts that were finally implanted was not affected by nicotine administration but the time of zona pellucida loss and growth of inner cell mass were delayed.

In a related study by Card and Mitchell (1978), administration of nicotine was shown to suppress uterine responsiveness by affecting the uterine lining so that it does not support implantation. The authors suggest that this decreased responsiveness may be due to nicotine-related alterations in ovarian steroid levels.

Maximal sensitivity of the uterus for implantation requires the presence of estrogen and progesterone in a ratio of 1:2000 ng. (Card & Mitchell, 1978). In this optimal ratio, estrogen potentiates the uterine sensitizing effect of progesterone. If estrogen levels are higher than those normally occurring in early pregnancy, estrogen exerts an inhibitory effect on uterine responsiveness to implantation (Card, 1978). Yoshinaga and his co-workers (1979) have in fact reported that nicotine alters the secretion of both estrogen and progesterone in early pregnancy. In control rats, serum progesterone levels were found to increase considerably during day 3 of pregnancy, whereas in nicotine-treated rats the increase was delayed by about 12 hours. This delay resulted in significantly lower progesterone levels in nicotine-treated animals at various times on gestation day 3. At the same time, serum estrogen levels in nicotine-treated animals were considerably higher compared to control animals. On the basis of these results, Yoshinaga concluded that the delay in implantation associated with nicotine administration is due to the suppression of progesterone secretion.

MENSTRUATION

Several studies have documented an earlier onset of menopause among women who smoke (Bailey *et al.*, 1977; Jick *et al.*, 1977; Kaufman *et al.*, 1980; Lindquist & Bengtsson, 1979; Daniell, 1978). This relationship is shown in Table 20 which presents the number of women at different ages who were postmenopausal on the basis of whether or not they were smokers. As indicated by the table, at each age there is a greater proportion of postmenopausal women among smokers as compared to non-smokers. Moreover, there is a dose-response relationship between the number of cigarettes smoked per day and the age of onset of menopause. For example, Kaufman and his co-workers (1980) reported onset of menopause at 49.4 years of age for nonsmokers, 48.0 years for women who smoked 1–14 cigarettes per day, and 47.6 years for women who smoked 15 or more cigarettes per day. Jick and co-workers (1977) found that between the ages of 44 and 53, only 35%

TABLE 20.   Relation between Smoking and Menopause[a]

Age (years)	Smoking status	Number of women	Number postmenopausal (%)
44–45	Smoker	366	47 (12.8%)
	Nonsmoker	366	44 (12.0%)
46–47	Smoker	350	107 (30.6%)
	Nonsmoker	327	75 (22.9%)
48–49	Smoker	385	172 (44.7%)
	Nonsmoker	322	122 (37.9%)
50–51	Smoker	344	251 (73.0%)
	Nonsmoker	384	247 (64.3%)
52–53	Smoker	334	291 (87.1%)
	Nonsmoker	354	275 (77.7%)

[a]Data from: Bailey *et al.*, 1977 and Jick *et al.*, 1977.

of the women studied (N = 2143) were postmenopausal among nonsmokers, whereas among those women who smoked one-half pack per day, there were 43% postmenopausal, and among those who smoked one or more packs per day, 49% were postmenopausal. Ex-smokers were found to be more likely menopausal than women who never smoked, but were less likely to be postmenopausal than current smokers.

Three possibilities have been suggested to account for this relation between smoking and earlier onset of menopause. The first is the "constitutionality hypothesis," whereby early menopause and smoking are both due to some other, as yet unidentified, physiological factor. This hypothesis is unlikely in light of the dose-response relation between smoking and menopause, the fact that this relation has been noted among women from several countries and different cultures, and the fact that ex-smokers are less likely to be postmenopausal than current smokers.

The second possibility is that earlier onset of menopause among smokers is due to their being less overweight than nonsmokers. Since obese women tend to have a later menopause, women who do not smoke would have a later onset of menopause due to their obesity. However, when women of the same weight were compared, smokers had an earlier age of onset than nonsmokers (Daniell, 1978).

The third possibility is that substances in tobacco smoke may affect ovarian enzymes or may destroy primordial oocytes. Menopause occurs when ovaries are depleted of oocytes and studies in mice have shown that benzo(a)pyrene is capable of oocyte destruction (Mattison & Thorgiersson, 1978). However, the large doses used in this study (20, 240 mg/kg) may not be relevant with respect to cigarette smoking among women.

Menstrual Disorders

Menstrual disorders associated with smoking have not been studied to any great extent. Wood and co-workers (1979a) did not find that women who smoked had longer or shorter menstrual cycles than nonsmokers, but in another study they reported that smokers were more likely to complain of menstrual pain than non-smokers. Premenstrual tension, however, was not related to smoking (Wood *et al.*, 1979b).

Summary and Conclusions

The evidence that smoking affects male libido is inconclusive. Studies in animals are also equivocal because of the possibility that decreases in sexual behavior may be due to secondary effects or to doses of drug that cause general malaise. While there is some evidence that smoking affects spermatogenesis, this is not the case for the overwhelming number of smokers. Sperm motility may be affected by smoking in some men, but not in most.

The female reproductive system seems much more sensitive to cigarette smoke and nicotine than the male's. Several studies have indicated that cigarette smoke or nicotine can affect the release of hormones involved in reproduction. In the case of luteinizing hormone, the site of action for this effect is not found in the pituitary but probably lies in the hypothalamus or higher cortical centers.

Studies of menopause are quite consistent in indicating an earlier onset of menopause in smokers compared to nonsmokers. The reason for this earlier onset has not yet been determined.

References

Bailey, A., Robinson, D., and Vessey, M. Smoking and age of natural menopause. *Lancet*, 1977, 2, 722.

Bignami, G. Pharmacologic influences on mating behavior in the male rat. Effects of D-amphetamine, LSD-25, strychnine, nicotine, and various anticholinergic agents. *Psychopharmacologia*, 1966, 10, 44–58.

Blake, C. A., Scaramuzzi, R. J., Norman, R. L., Kanematsu, S., and Sawyer, C. H. Nicotine delays the ovulatory surge of luteinizing hormone in the rat. *Proceedings of the Society for Experimental Biology and Medicine*, 1972a, 141, 1014–1016.

Blake, C. A., Scaramuzzi, R. J., Norman, R. L., Kanematsu, S., and Sawyer, C. H. Effect of nicotine on the proestrous ovulatory surge of LH in the rat. *Endocrinology*, 1972b, 91, 1253–1258.

Blake, C. A. and Sawyer, C. H. Nicotine blocks the suckling-induced rise in circulating prolactin in lactating rats. *Science*, 1972c, *177*, 619–621.

Blake, C. A., Norman, R. L., Scaramuzzi, R. J., and Sawyer, C. H. Inhibition of the proestrous surge of prolactin in the rat by nicotine. *Endocrinology*, 1972d, *91*, 1334–1338.

Blake, C. A. Parallelism and divergence in luteinizing hormone and follicle stimulating hormone release in nicotine-treated rats. *Proceedings of the Society for Experimental Biology and Medicine*, 1974, *145*, 716–720.

Briggs, M. H. Cigarette smoking and infertility in men. *Medical Journal of Australia*, 1973, *7*, 616–617.

Brooks, J. E. *Tobacco, its history illustrated by the books, manuscripts and engravings in the library of George Arents, Jr., together with an introductory essay, a glossary, and bibliographic notes.* 1937, Vol. 1, 1507–1615. New York: The Rosenbach Company.

Campbell, J. M. and Harrison, K. L. Smoking and infertility. *Medical Journal of Australia*, 1979, *1*, 342–343.

Card, J. P. and Mitchell, J. A. The effects of nicotine administration on deciduoma induction in the rat. *Biology of Reproduction*, 1978, *19*, 326–331.

Card, J. P. and Mithcell, J. A. Effects of nicotine on implantation in the rat. *Biology of Reproduction*, 1979, *20*, 532–539.

Cattanach, B. M. Lack of effect of nicotine on the fertility of male and female mice. *Zeitschrift fur Vererbungslehre*, 1962, *93*, 351–355.

Cendron, H. and Vallery-Masson, J. Les effets de L'age sur l'activite sexuelle masculine. Incidences de quelques facteurs dont le tabac. *La Presse Medicale*, 1970, *78*, 1795–1797.

Daniell, H. W. Smoking, obesity, and the menopause. *Lancet*, 1978, *2*, 373.

Dontewill, W., Chevalier, H. J., Harke, H. P., Lafrenz, U., Rechzeh, G., and Schneider, B. Experimental investigations of the effect of cigarette smoke exposure on testicular function of syrian golden hamsters. *Toxicology*, 1973, *1*, 309–320.

Eneroth, P., Fuxe, K., Gustafsson, J. A., Hokfelt, T., Lofstrom, A., Skett, P., and Agnati, L. The effect of nicotine on central catecholamine neurons and gonadotropin secretion. II. Inhibitory influence of nicotine on LH, FSH, and prolactin secretion in the ovariectomized female rat and its relation to regional changes in dopamine and noradrenaline levels and turnover. *Medical Biology*, 1977, *55*, 158–166.

Eneroth, P., Fuxe, K., Gustafsson, J. A., Hokfelt, T., Lofstrom, A., Skett, P., and Agnati, L. The effect of nicotine on central catecholamine neurons and gonadotropin secretion. III. Studies on prepubertal female rats treated with pregnant mare serum gonadotropin. *Medical Biology*, 1977, *55*, 167–176.

Erbacher, K., Grumbrecht, P., and Loser, A. Nikotin und inners sekretion. *Archiv fur experimentelle pathologie und pharmakologie*, 1940, *195*, 121–141.

Evans, H. J., Fletcher, J., Torrance, M., and Hargreave, T. B. Sperm abnormalities and cigarette smoking. *Lancet*, 1981, *1*, 627–629.

Ferry, J. D., McLean, B. K., and Nikitovitch-Winer, M. B. Tobacco-smoke inhalation delays suckling-induced prolactin release in the rat. *Proceedings of the Society for Experimental Biology and Medicine*, 1974, *147*, 110–113.

Forsberg, L., Gustavii, B., Hojerback, T., and Olsson, A. M. Impotence, smoking, and blocking Drugs. *Fertility and Sterility*, 1979, *31*, 589–591.

Fuxe, K., Agnati, L., Eneroth, P., Gustafsson, J. A., Hokfelt, T., Lofstrom, A., Skett, B., and Skett, P. The effect of nicotine on central catecholamine neurons and gonadotropin secretion. I. Studies in the male rat. *Medical Biology*, 1977, *55*, 148–157.

Fuxe, K., Everitt, B. J., and Hokfelt, T. Enhancement of sexual behavior in the female rat by nicotine. *Pharmacology, Biochemistry, and Behavior*, 1977, *7*, 147–151.

Godfrey, B. Sperm morphology in smokers. *Lancet*, 1981, *1*, 948.

Hammond, E. C. Smoking in relation to physical complaints. *Archives of Environmental Health*, 1961, *3*, 28–46.

Hamor, R. *A true discourse of the present estate of virginia*. London, 1615. Repr. in *The historie of travile into virginia britannia* R. H, Major (ed.), London: Hakluyt Soc., 1849.

Hollick, F. H. *The marriage guide*, New York, 1850.

Jick, H., Porter, J., and Morrison, A. S. Relation between smoking and age of natural menopause. Report from the Boston Collaborative Drug Surveillance Program, Boston University Medical Center. *Lancet*, 1977, *1*, 1354.

Kaufman, D. W., Slone, D., Rosenberg, L., Miettinen, O. S., and Shapiro, S. Cigarette smoking and age at natural menopause. *American Journal of Public Health*, 1980, *70*, 420–422.

Lall, K. B., Singhi, S., Gurnani, M., Singhi, P., and Garg, O. P. Somatotype, physical growth, and sexual maturation in young male smokers. *Journal of Epidemiology and Community Health*, 1980, *34*, 295–298.

Larson, P. S., Haag, H. B., and Silvette, H. *Tobacco, experimental and clinical studies: A comprehensive account of the world literature*. Baltimore, Maryland, Williams and Wilkins Co., 1961.

Lindquist, O. and Bengtsson, C. Menopausal age in relation to smoking. *Acta Medica Scandinavica*, 1979, *205*, 73–77.

Longo, F. J. and Anderson, E. The effects of nicotine on fertilization in the sea urchin, *Arbacia Punctulata*. *Journal of Cell Biology*, 1970, *46*, 308–325.

Malcolm, S. and Shephard, R. J. Personality and sexual behavior of the adolescent smoker. *American Journal of Drug and Alcohol Abuse*, 1978, *5*, 87–96.

Mattison, D. R. and Thorgiersson, S. S. Smoking and industrial pollution, and their effects on menopause and ovarian cancer. *Lancet*, 1978, *1*, 187–188.

Maynwaring, E. *Morbus Polyrhizos and Polymorphaeus*. London, 1669.

McLean, B. K., Rubel, A., and Nikitovitch-Winer, M. B. The differential effects of exposure to tobacco smoke on the secretion of luteinizing hormone and prolactin in the proestrous rat. *Endocrinology*, 1977, *100*, 1566–1570.

Mellan, J. Smoking and male sexual defects. *Prakticke Zubni Lekarstvi*, 1963, *43*, 862–863.

Neri, A. and Marcus, S. L. Effect of nicotine on the motility of the oviducts in the rhesus monkey: A preliminary report. *Journal of Reproduction and Fertility*, 1972, *31*, 91–97.

Ochsner, A. Influence of smoking on sexuality and pregnancy. *Medical Aspects of Human Sexuality*, 1977, *5*, 78–92.

Persky, H., O'Brian, C. P., Fine, E., Howard, W. J., Kahn, M. A., and Beck, R. W. The effect of alcohol and smoking on testicular function and aggression in chronic alcoholics. *American Journal of Psychiatry*, 1977, *134*, 621–625.

Pettersson, F., Fries, H., and Nillius, S. J. Epidemiology of secondary amenorrhea. I. Incidence and prevalence rates. *American Journal of Obstetrics and Gynecology*, 1973, *117*, 80–86.

Philaretes. *Work for chimney-sweepers*. London, 1601–1602. Repr. by Shakespear Assoc., London, Oxford University Press, 1936.

Phillips, L. G. Cigarette smoking as a factor in sterility. *Hawaii Medical Journal*, 1943, *2*, 249.

Raboch, J. and Mellan, J. Smoking and fertility. *British Journal of Sexual Medicine*, 1975, *2*, 35–36.

Schirren, C. Die kinderlose ehe. Moglichkeiten und grenzen der behandlung aus andrologischer sichts. *Fortschritte der Medizin*, 1970, *24*, 1047–1051.

Schirren, C. Die wirkung des nikotins auf die zeugungsfahigkeit des mannes. *Rehabilitation*, 1972, *25*, 23–24.

Seltzer, C. C. Masculinity and smoking. *Science*, 1959, *130*, 1706–1707.

Soulairac, M. L. and Soulairac, A. Action de la nicotine sur le comportement sexuel du rat male. *Comptes Rendus de Seance de la Societé de Biologie et Medicine*, 1972, *166*, 798–802.

Stadtlander, K. H. Uber die wirkung des nikotins auf reimdrusen und nebennieren. *Zeitschrift fur die gesamte experimentelle medizin*, 1936, *99*, 670–680.

Sterling, T. D. and Kobayashi, D. A critical review of reports on the effect of smoking on sex and fertility. *Journal of Sex Research*, 1975, *11*, 201–217.

Subak-Sharpe, G. J. Is your sex life going up in smoke? *Today's Health*, 1974, *52*, 50–53.

Tokuhata, G. Smoking in relation to infertility and fetal loss. *Archives of Environmental Health*, 1968, *17*, 353–359.

Vessey, M. P., Wright, N. H., McPherson, K., and Wiggins, P. Fertility after stopping different methods of contraception. *British Medical Journal*, 1978, *1*, 265–267.

Viczian, M. The effect of cigarette smoke inhalation on spermatogenesis in rats. *Experientia*, 1968, *24*, 511–512.

Wilson, R. H., McNaught, J. N., and Deeds, F. Chronic nicotine toxicity. IV. Effect of nicotin-containing diets on histology and weights of organs of albino rats. *Journal of Industrial Hygiene and Toxicology*, 1937, *20*, 468–481.

Winternitz, W. W. and Quillen, D. Acute hormonal response to cigarette smoking. *Journal of Clinical Pharmacology*, 1977, *134*, 621–625.

Wood, C., Larsen, L. and Williams, R. Duration of menstruation. *Australian and New Zealand Journal of Obstetrics and Gynaecology*, 1979, *19*, 216–219.

Wood, C., Larsen, L. and Williams, R. Social and psychological factors in relation to premenstrual tension and menstrual pain. *Australian and New Zealand Journal of Obstetrics and Gynaecology*, 1979, *19*, 111–115.

Yoshinaga, K., Rice, C., Krenn, J., and Pilot, R. L. Effects of nicotine on early pregnancy in the rat. *Biology of Reproduction*, 1979, *20*, 294–303.

Index

229